Girl, Put on Your Lipstick—

THE
WORLD
NEEDS
YOU

*A Guide to Living Unapologetically and
Authentically in Your 40s and Beyond*

LAUREN HALE

Girl, Put on Your Lipstick—The World Needs You
A Guide to Living Unapologetically and Authentically in Your 40s and Beyond
Lauren Hale

Copyright © 2025 - Reflek Publishing

For more information: lauren.hale2@gmail.com

ISBN PAPERBACK: 978-1-962280-76-1

ISBN EBOOK: 978-1-962280-77-8

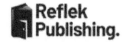
Reflek Publishing.

Dedication

To my children:

I wrote this book for you. My hope is that you will always follow your dreams. Wherever they may take you. No dream is too big or too impossible. Life isn't about following the crowd; it is about standing out and following your heart. Someday, I hope you look at yourselves and are truly proud of your journey. The ups and the downs. The good times and the hard times, know that all of those experiences were molding you into the person you have become.

I love you always,

Mom

Table of Contents

Introduction

As a young girl, I always believed I could do or be anything. I would spend hours talking to myself in the mirror, accepting pretend awards and dreaming one day about being "someone."

I wasn't someone special. I had no big "gifts." I wasn't top in my class. I wasn't a great singer. I wasn't the most popular. I was honestly just "average." I always had to work really hard to get good grades. In sports, I was never extraordinary. I had to put in twice the effort as my peers to be even half as good as them. The one thing I had going for me was determination.

I knew if I wanted something, I could go after it. I always did whatever it took to get there, and I didn't always get where I wanted, but my crazy brain would say, *keep going, Lauren!*

That determined little girl started to grow up. She traded her Lip Smackers for sparkly gloss, and somewhere between believing in Santa Claus and middle school she began thinking she wasn't good enough. I forgot the girl that thought she could rule the world and I started to lose myself. It wasn't until my 40s that I slowly began to find my spark again. I found myself again and re-embraced all the things that bring me joy. Rediscovering myself was a process of re-learning who I am, and I hope that I can share with you some of the ways I did that in hopes that you can find yourself again too.

At age 40, something clicked in me. I was tired of living my life for others. I was tired of just fitting in and I was exhausted from people-pleasing. I was living my life for others and in the process of doing that, I had lost who I was.

To be honest, I was ready to give up. I felt like I had changed myself so many times for others, that I didn't know who I was anymore or what I even liked. I was living a life where I just wanted others to like me so badly, that I didn't even like myself anymore.

I was depressed and alone and that feeling was something I know many of you have experienced or are experiencing now. It's a horrible feeling. I was at my lowest point, but no one on the outside would know because I just kept smiling. It was almost like if I pretended everything was okay, no one would know my brokenness.

The sad thing is, so many of us do this. We pretend we are okay. We pretend we love our lives, even though some days we can hardly get out of bed. We pretend to be happy. I finally decided that this wasn't how I wanted to live anymore. One day, I just got tired of pretending. I didn't want to be the person people wanted me to be. I wanted to actually live life on my own terms.

Maybe you can relate. I promise you it isn't always easy, but you can change your circumstances. You can find your joy again. You can start living a life that you want. You can drown out the noise, and you can choose to change your life, no matter your age. This book will help you change the narrative and learn to make decisions on how you can start living a life that you want and stop living for others. This book is going to help you find that spark you once had.

It starts with a yes. It starts with setting boundaries and it starts with putting in the work, which I will talk about in the following chapters, to start fully loving yourself for who you are. The challenging days will make you stronger and the good days will help you see how far you have come. It might be hard to see that right now but throughout this book I will share examples of how I became grateful for the hard days and how they changed me.

I found, after doing lots of soul searching, that the stories we tell ourselves matter. They create our inner voice. And our inner voice is often doubtful, critical, and insecure. It's so loud and demanding that the stories we told ourselves through childhood—the ones that said we could be CEOs and princesses and joyful moms—begin to change. Now we're worrying about failing. People liking us. Having regrets. Making mistakes. We're writing tragedies in the lines where we used to daydream—but all of this can change. We can change the stories we tell ourselves—again—and write new ones that encourage us to keep going. Those mistakes we were once afraid of are actually huge steps in the journey of finding ourselves.

The truth is, the stories we tell ourselves can make or break us. We can choose to focus on the stories of our setbacks or grief or our hard past. . .or we can focus on the stories of when we have overcome. We can start changing the narrative at any time and write a new one.

This book is about writing a new story as we age. We are not our past, and we can still find our joy. Your age doesn't matter, and you are never too old to change. You can always write a new chapter. You are not stuck.

Little did I know that playing with makeup and taking selfies would lead me to a journey of finding myself again, and I can't wait to share how you can begin to write a new chapter too.

Makeup Mini-Tutorial: Plot Lines Change

We all have a story to tell. This is the story of how I started over when I didn't think I could. I thought I was "too old" to try something new. I left my teaching career, feeling burned out and exhausted, and rewrote my story. This is my journey of starting over at 40 and how I became a makeup influencer who has touched thousands of women's lives in the process.

https://www.instagram.com/p/C4HSdgtR0RJ/

Chapter One

Change

*Only I can change my life. No one can do it for
me.*

— Carol Burnett

*If you truly want to change your life, you must
first be willing to change your mind.*

— Donald Altman

I felt a sense of uncertainty as I looked into the now empty
Kindergarten classroom that was only a few days ago was filled
with laughter, bright posters, encouraging sayings, and kids'
artwork. This room that once held so many memories was now
dark and empty. Boxes packed with my old teaching materials—
materials that I worked so hard to get—took the place of the
tables, chairs and cubbies filled with backpacks and lunchboxes
that once lined the walls. This was my home for five years. But
with anything, a new chapter requires turning the page to get
to the new one. As I looked back one more time, I flicked off the

light and closed the heavy door behind me, ready to embrace this new chapter of life.

Five years earlier, in 2011, I was a 35-year-old stay at home mom, with three kids under the age of eight. Don't get me wrong, I loved my life, but I needed more. I had gone to school for many years to secure my teaching degree, and before I had kids, I worked with children who had special needs. Once I had my kids, I decided the best place for me was to be home with them—especially when they were young. I always planned to go back to teaching, eventually. Eight years later, my kids were all in school and I was wondering whether it was time for me to return to the classroom myself. That's when I received a phone call about an opening for a Kindergarten teaching job at a private Christian school in town. They told me if I took that job that my kids could also attend school while I worked. So of course I said yes! For the next five years, I spent my time teaching five-year-olds how to read and how to write their names. It was my dream job. Those kids changed me. They gave me back my light, they made me laugh, and they brought out my creativity I had lost for so long. I *loved* my job, and I worked with the best people, but after five years, my life began to change. I began to change. I knew another chapter in my life was coming to a close, and that there was more for me out there.

And just like that, I was changing my life again. I left a job I thought I would never leave. A job that brought me so much, but I had changed. I needed more and I took the chance to walk away even though I had received so much joy from teaching. I just felt like something was missing.

Have you ever felt a calling for more. . . like life isn't done with you just yet? I believe we all have a path, a journey in life that we are meant for; we just have to listen to that voice and go after it even when we feel scared. Even when we feel like it's a scary move to make. I promise if you listen to that voice, change can happen. It doesn't matter your age, your background, or your situation because I believe if you listen to that voice it will take you to greatness. It will lead you to the life you were meant for.

You see, change begins the moment you are willing to go after what you want. At 39, I loved what I was doing, but I also felt pulled in so many directions as a mom. I felt burned out. I was spending long hours away from my family working in a classroom with other people's kids, writing lesson plans on the weekends, and worrying about how I was going to find a substitute to teach my class when one of my babies woke up sick. I was exhausted with life. My husband was working long hours to pay bills, and my teaching salary was not making sense to spend the hours away from my family.

COVID-19 was my breaking point. I was working online, writing lesson plans online, and doing Google Meets with Kindergarteners (I'm sure you can imagine the things I saw), all while teaching my own kids at home. It was a lot!

The next year when we were allowed to go back to school, we went back with masks. Let's just say Kindergarteners wearing masks was so hard. Five-year-olds communicate and learn through expression, and wearing a mask was something that they struggled with, especially when trying to learn to read and socialize with each other. Teaching reading to them with masks was almost impossible and looking around my room filled with Clorox wipes and plastic dividers made me sad. Trying to teach them social skills and keep normalcy all while having to sanitize and meet protocols started to drain me.

The girl who used to love going to work slowly started to dread it. If you have ever felt dread about doing something, you know what I mean. I knew I needed to change my life. I knew it wasn't fair to myself but also to the kids in my classroom. I started to feel like I wasn't present and the joy I used to have just wasn't there anymore.

You Have to Be Willing

The first part with change is you have to want it and you have to be willing. It doesn't matter how scared you are. Take that piece out, because you will always be scared, but if you want change you will do it anyway. You have to be willing to change how you are living your life. You have to be so tired of the way you are living to finally say, "I've had enough." If you are struggling with change, you are not lazy, you are just *unwilling* to change. We get so set in our daily routines, even though we may hate them, it's sometimes easier to go on cruise control than face reality. The reality that we truly aren't happy. Ask yourself, are you willing to stay in that relationship? Are you willing to stay unhealthy? Are you willing to keep working 60 to 70 hours a week?

When you decide what you are willing to handle and take on, that's where you discover your full potential. When you make a conscious choice to face whatever challenges and responsibilities may arise, you are more prepared to accept them. The more you are open to taking on new challenges and confronting difficulties, the more you can grow and reach your true potential.

In order to truly be willing to change, you have to be so unhappy with the life you are living that you want to create a new one. And here's the thing: you can always start over. You can always create a new path. The first step is wanting to change your story. You have to want to create a new script. You have to want to create a new version of yourself. This new version is you chasing your dreams and living the life you have always wanted for yourself, because you can. Life is too short to sit back and not live. You were made for something so much bigger, but it's up to you to actually pivot. It's up to you to want something so bad, that nothing or no one will stop you from living a life you deserve or want for yourself.

When I was working as a teacher, even though I loved it, I knew I wanted more. I would spend my summers selling teaching materials, hosting Kindergarten learning programs and taking extra courses to be a more innovative educator. The problem for me is all of this still took me away from my family. I didn't understand why I couldn't have both. Why couldn't I be a present mom but also have something for myself? It was a thought I wrestled with for a long time.

When you are looking to change anything in life, the biggest factor is belief. There have been many times in my life when I've felt self-doubt creep in. It feels like a loud voice in my head telling me "I'm too old to change," "I'm not pretty enough," or "I'm not smart enough to do that." Even the people around me have caused self-doubt; we will talk more in another chapter about how to get those people out of your life or at least silence that noise.

In fact, the people telling you that you can't do something are probably the same people that aren't willing to change their own situation. Self-doubt kills your dreams. It stalls you from taking that first leap toward change. When you doubt yourself, it's really hard to have confidence in your mission or what you are doing. Our fears are learned. We all have stories that have gotten us to where we are today. We all have had people put beliefs into us, good or bad. Our fears and self-doubt are all learned, and those deep-rooted fears never go away by ignoring them. We have to learn to face them head on.

A lot of times, it isn't just self-doubt that kills our dreams, it is external doubt. External doubt can come from someone on the outside that is important to you, or who had a role in your life that meant something. Perhaps a parent criticized you, a teacher voiced a concern that didn't seem valid, or a close friend said something that caused you to doubt yourself or what you were doing. Comments made by people who are close to us tend to hit harder, don't they? Know this: Not everyone is going to agree with you. When you know where your values lie, you can choose to think for yourself and face fear head on.

I've been trying to prove myself from the moment I arrived on this earth as a preemie. My mom always said I couldn't get here soon enough, that I came out and hit the ground running. I started walking before nine months old, I was reading novels like the old Nancy Drew books before I was eight, and I always had this drive to find recognition for tasks I was "good at."

But all of this proving myself taught me that I wasn't enough. I truly felt that if I wasn't number one at something, I was inadequate. I was born with a perfectionist and competitive internal drive to constantly be the best at everything I did. My parents and coaches were never the ones doubting me; it was always this internal struggle and pressure from myself to be seen. Most of my doubt came from my own thoughts of not being good enough. They came from the need for others to recognize my accomplishments and what I was doing. I led my life like this for many years and always felt that if I wasn't getting recognized I wasn't doing "well enough." It was not until years later that I understood what I was doing to myself and had to work on changing the way my thought patterns had been developed.

Thinking this way led to years of anxiety, doubt and trying to prove to everyone around me that I was extraordinary. I realized later that it never mattered what others thought; it was how I saw myself that mattered. I had to learn how to reverse the perception I had of myself.

The problem with this is that not only is it exhausting, but you will never prove to anyone you are good enough. Despite what anyone says, it will never change how you think or feel about yourself. When you don't truly believe in yourself, it doesn't matter how many people believe in you. It starts with *you*. You can be told over and over by others how incredible or exceptional you are, but if you don't actually believe it, those words take on no meaning for you. You have to prove it to yourself. You have to stop trying to make others see your potential, and start seeing it for yourself.

As children, we are so curious. We are willing to take risks. We don't even think about failing or how we look to others. As we get older, we start to lose our curiosity and begin to fear trying new things. We start telling ourselves stories and make up "what if" situations that hold us back. We're born curious, but external situations slowly chip away at our curiosity, leaving us with the belief that we aren't allowed to ask questions. We can't wonder what life we could have if only we asked questions and were brave. Instead, we remember the last time we failed at something. We couldn't possibly try anything new again. We hold onto critical remarks that no one else even remembers. Our minds are powerful, and they can change as we grow. For worse. . . or for better.

What it really comes down to is fear and belief. If we believe we aren't enough, then we fear failure. Because the only way we can be enough is to succeed. If we think about it, what we really fear is what others will think of us if we do fail. And more than that, we fear what we will think of ourselves. It's all a part of this belief system we've crafted since adolescence and the stories we tell ourselves.

When I was a little girl, I would dive into any situation with a fury. I wanted to conquer life and didn't even understand what "failing" meant. The fear of failure started for me in elementary school. We moved to a new state when I was in fourth grade; I didn't know anyone and wanted to make friends and fit in. I wanted to be liked, and I never wanted my teachers or my parents to think less of me. I strived to be seen as the daughter or student who followed the rules, was a good girl, and who helped the teacher. I never liked being in trouble, so I learned to play it safe. I learned that doing what adults asked of me made me be more acknowledged and accepted. The less curious I was, the more I fit in and others liked me. I was the girl that could fit into a group, but kids my age didn't always notice I was there. I became really good at morphing into an image that others wanted me to be.

It wasn't until my 40s that I started giving myself permission to fail. By fail, I mean trying things that I wasn't necessarily good at but was curious if I could do it. I attempted kayaking, cliff jumping, riding roller coasters even though I was scared of heights, playing pickleball, and joining a women's tennis league (even though college had burned me out). I wasn't horrible at these things, and I loved seeing if I could do it. I loved the feeling of moving my body or learning a new skill. The more I tried things out of my comfort zone, the more I realized that I didn't have to be perfect or the best at everything. I began to see that failing wasn't bad or wrong, but instead saw that life gives you what you need. Trying things out of my comfort zone, doing something I wasn't good at right away taught me that I could try new things and learn about myself through the process. The more uncomfortable or challenged I was, the more I learned that when things don't turn out how you want or expect, what I thought was a roadblock was actually just a detour taking me to where I was supposed to be.

Failure isn't something to be scared of because you can't actually fail—you can only learn. Setbacks teach us lessons and carry us closer to our dreams. As kids, we didn't even realize we were "failing" unless we got a bad grade, our friends made fun of us, or we didn't read enough books that summer to get a free personal pan pizza from Pizza Hut. But once we realized failure was a thing that could happen to us, we started listening to what others thought of us and began rewriting the stories we told ourselves. And just like that, we changed our beliefs. We began to believe failure was a bad thing, and one that must be avoided at all costs. So at the cost of ensuring we never failed, we stopped giving ourselves permission to try.

After finally learning to give myself grace through failure, I began to realize I was the only one who could change. It wasn't about what others thought of me. It wasn't about how good I was at something. It was all about what I believed about myself. It was my ability to start taking risks, believing in myself and realizing that the only person that needed to believe in me was *me.*

Even while I was going through change, I was still dealing with the fear of not being good enough, and yes, even the fear of failing. Despite these fears, I had to have the courage to make a change or be okay with staying with where I was. It took changing my own mindset to rewrite my story. It takes one thought. One first step. It takes rewiring your brain to believe that you have the ability to change your life. The only person that can do that is you.

Know Your Why

So, why do you want to make a change? Our minds tend to focus on the things we think we want, but a lot of times we aren't willing to make the changes it takes to get there. So where do you begin? Begin today. Take those small steps toward change. Map out the strategies you need to change. What is it going to take? Once you answer these questions, then just start. It really is that simple. Want to lose weight? Start moving. Don't want to go to the gym? Eat less or take that extra walk during the day. If you don't want to do those things, then maybe this isn't really a goal you want.

Stop pretending to yourself you want something unless you are actually willing to change to get it. It will not be easy. If you decide along the way that you don't really want something, give yourself grace while trying to figure out what you actually do want.

Sometimes when you think you want to change something and then realize it isn't something you are truly willing to put the work into evolving, you learn more about yourself. This is all part of the process. When you stop lying to yourself about what you want it actually becomes freeing.

As you are working toward your goals, thoughts you believe about yourself will start popping into your head. Thoughts like, *I weigh too much because I'm lazy* or *I'm a failure because I tried this business and didn't sell anything.* Feel those thoughts. Are they true or are you identifying from your past? The future you is ready for change, so could your results be different this time?

Of course! Changing your mindset to the here and now instead of results-based thinking changes everything.

It takes resilience and consistency to change. You may start something and realize it isn't for you. Even if it is the path you are supposed to take, you may not find success right away, but you will learn a lot about yourself along the way. There will be ups and downs. Change isn't always easy. It comes slowly, and you will oftentimes find there are more lows than highs along the way.

Lean into that self-growth. Allow yourself to show up as fully as you. Be consistent. Don't give up, even when you really want to. To give whatever you are going after your absolute all, that is when you will start to see change and success.

When you lean into the hard, it will challenge your beliefs about yourself. A lot of us have "traumas" that we need to work through. We have stories we have told ourselves that we must rewrite. We may need to be placed in uncomfortable situations so we can continue to challenge our beliefs.

Change takes time. It isn't easy, but once you start taking those small steps, you will be surprised at how your life starts changing too. Those small steps won't happen overnight. For example, let's say you hate your job and want to find a new one. Maybe you can't afford to just quit right away. Big changes don't always have lasting results. Quitting the job you hate and not having an income will quite possibly backfire on you and you may end up in financial distress.

A small step might be looking at your expenses and seeing where you can cut back so you can save money, so when you do transition to a new job the financial burden will be easier. Those small changes help you plan for the changes you ultimately want to make in your life.

That doesn't mean you can't give those small steps your all. Consistency, determination, and grit are all necessary to make the changes, big or small, you need to make in order to get the life you want.

Sometimes you know you need change, but you don't even know where to start.

One example of change in my life was when I became a mom for the first time. I remember being so excited when I found out I was pregnant and I started to imagine what this new life was going to look like with our new baby. When my son was born, it actually wasn't anything like I had romanticized in my mind. Instead of loving every minute, I often felt resentful and even sad. As much as I loved this new baby more than anything in the entire world, I realized my freedom and the life I knew had changed. I remember being at such a low, sitting by myself while my new baby slept in the other room. I would just cry. I felt alone and isolated. This new life wasn't what I had imagined. I doubted myself and felt so scared that I was in charge of this little person. Could I be the mom I wanted to be? How was I going to protect this baby and give him the life he deserved? What if I did something wrong? These questions were constantly circling in my brain.

There is always the possibility you will doubt yourself when you enter change, even if it's something you want. Your mind is powerful and the thoughts you feed it will grow. You can feel lost and still be changing. It's a process of discovering yourself. It's not always easy. It took time to feel like I was capable of being a mom. Learning how to change tiny diapers, correctly install a car seat, and understanding how to get my son on a good feeding and sleeping schedule, all took time. It wasn't something that happened right away. I read a lot of books. I asked other more experienced moms for advice and I leaned on my own mom a lot too for her help. It was those small action steps that I took that got me started and overtime taught me to have confidence in my parenting skills.

When you get clarity on what you really want, a whole new world will open up for you. Clarity doesn't happen overnight. It ultimately begins with you looking for answers. Sometimes it looks like asking someone more experienced, and sometimes it looks like you taking a chance and trying your own way. It really is all about experimenting to see what works; and sometimes when you find what works you may have to pivot again. The more you keep trying, the more you will gain clarity on what you want and what works.

So here's the big question: are you really ready to change your life? If so, start paying close attention to your thought patterns. Listen to how you talk to yourself—what you say out loud about yourself to others. Words are powerful, and we believe the stories we tell ourselves. When you find yourself thinking or saying thoughts that aren't serving you, try to rephrase them in a different way. An example might be, "I'm not very good at that." A way to rephrase that could be, "I'm not good at that yet, but I am working hard to improve." Rewiring your thought patterns can be so powerful. When you change your thoughts, you change your world.

Action steps for change:

1. Identify what area in your life you want to change. What are you unhappy with? Where do you feel like you are being held back? Identify what you want to change and then decide if you are truly ready to change your situation. It helps to write it all down on paper so you can visualize and gain clarity. And if you realize you don't really want the change you thought you did, that's okay. You're not a failure for not wanting that change.

2. Have a support system. Surround yourself with others who want you to succeed, who see your goals and want to support you. Have them hold you accountable.

3. Take baby steps. Make a plan. What are the action steps you need to start now to achieve your vision? Write down the first small step, then break it down into achievable bite-size pieces, and then begin. It's that easy!

4. Give yourself grace. You will not see success right away and you will become frustrated. Celebrate the small wins as you see progress. This will keep you going. It's sometimes hard to celebrate yourself, but the more you do the more you realize the greatness in what you are trying to achieve!

Journal Questions

1. How do I usually respond to change? Do I embrace or resist it?
2. How has a time in my life where I have had to change helped me grow as a person?
3. What fears do I have when I think about changing a part of my life that I am not happy with?

_____

_____

_____

_____

_____

_____

_____

_____

_____

_____

_____

_____

_____

_____

_____

_____

_____

_____

_____

_____

Makeup Mini-Tutorial: Applying Makeup Over 40 vs. The Old Way

As we age, our skin changes and our makeup should too. If you've begun to notice fine lines and wrinkles, texture, loose skin and more...relax. This is normal. Because of these new beauty marks on our face, many of us stop loving how makeup looks as we age. So, we stop wearing it altogether. With just a few tweaks though, I'll show you how you can start loving the way makeup looks on you again!

https://www.instagram.com/p/DAdxOeHvzuW/

Chapter Two

Setting Boundaries

Daring to set boundaries is about having the courage to love ourselves even when we risk disappointing others.

—Brené Brown

Setting boundaries has never come easy for me. I am a people pleaser to a fault. I thought that being a good friend, a good teammate or even a good family member meant saying "yes" and doing whatever people asked of me. In fact, in college at the ripe old age of nineteen I met my future husband on a blind date that I felt I couldn't say no to. We were actually set up by two of our college friends, who were currently dating and I am sure they just wanted another couple to hang out with. Either way, being the people-pleaser that I was, I said yes.

When I met my husband Nic, I remember getting out of the car to meet him. All five feet two inches and 100 pounds of me looked up at this big six foot-one 230-pound football player, wearing Wranglers, cowboy boots and a big Nebraska Cornhuskers belt buckle. We couldn't have been more different. But when I met him, I knew I wanted to see more of that cute, blonde-haired guy, so I tried really hard to make a good first impression. Even if that first impression meant telling a few "white lies." I figured until he got to know me, I would just answer his questions in a way that he would want a second date and later on (if it worked out) I would then be my real self.

I don't remember much about that night, but I do know I was super nervous and we hardly talked. I felt like he was interviewing me with his questions. One of them was, "Do you like rap music?" I knew this country boy did not like rap at all, so I replied, "No, just country." The truth was I warmed up to rap music whenever I played tennis and at that time in my life had never even heard a country song.

Luckily for me, my white lies did not trip up our relationship and after months of dating, we fell head over heels in love. When I was finally comfortable enough to let my true personality and strong-willed nature come out, he loved me all the more for them. Looking back, I realize how ridiculous this whole story sounds, but I'm sure you have done similar things to make others like you or to fit in with a friend group. Why do we spend so much of our lives trying to make others like us, being something we're not just so we can feel accepted?

Eventually, as I said, I did learn to state my opinions, likes and dislikes, but at the time I was so scared of people abandoning me if I did show the real me. I learned to become a chameleon, changing colors for different people and groups I was with. It was exhausting.

Years later, I did a deep dive into why I people-pleased and why I had a sense of abandonment and I realized that in the past anytime I had been myself around a guy or even a "best friend," (and I say that in quotation marks because they weren't really my friends) they would ditch me for another girl or leave me out of the group of friends or any other scenario you could imagine. I became so set on this story, that I truly believed that I had to be someone else in order to be liked. This story lived with me for many years.

We all have our own stories. Stories we tell ourselves based on past experiences, friends that have walked away, or romantic relationships that ended. We love to hold on to the stories we tell ourselves, almost like a badge of honor. We claim that this is who we are and we become stuck. What we don't realize is letting go of these stories is actually incredibly freeing. When we release them, we work our way out of the cocoon we should have left long ago and finally become the butterfly we always knew we were—what we were always meant to be.

Take it from me, a self-proclaimed recovering people-pleaser: life is too short to waste time doing things for the sake of doing things. Life is too short to do things that don't bring you joy. Life is too short to stay with people who want to "use" you. When you learn to set boundaries and how to say no you are giving yourself permission to find joy in what you want to find joy in. Learning to set boundaries with people isn't about being unkind—it's about respecting yourself enough to know what you can handle.

For me, I know I can't handle having "friends" in my life that are demanding of my time. My priorities right now are being a mom and a wife and the friend part comes last. I also have learned to set boundaries with my work. I used to work until all hours of the night, and since I work on my phone I would never put it down. It was interrupting family time and I was never "walking away" from work. I finally set hours for myself when I am off my phone. If someone doesn't respect that or like that, they are not someone I will work with anymore. If you can't handle something, and it isn't bringing you joy, it's time to move on and find what does.

Struggling To Set Boundaries

As long as I can remember, I have always struggled to set boundaries in my friendships, probably stemming from my desire to feel accepted. I struggled tremendously with wanting to fit in and never quite feeling like I did. I would somehow find myself in circles of women who would talk about you as soon as you left the room. They would leave me out, gossip about me and when I finally got the nerve up to confront them, they would say it was their duty to share the secret I had told them. No apologies, just me feeling once again abandoned and alone. All because I didn't know how to set boundaries. I let these so-called friends run all over me. I never spoke up when they hurt me, and by being silent I let it happen again and again, continuing to allow them to disrupt my peace.

Once I learned how to set boundaries, my circle grew smaller, but my friendships got tighter. I set boundaries by speaking up and verbalizing what I didn't like. I stopped doing things for others if it wasn't something that brought me joy. I confronted situations that I used to sit back and feel hurt by. I stopped pretending to be like them. I didn't want to be a part of a group where gossiping was normal. When I started sticking up for myself and setting boundaries, I lost a lot of these "friends." You have to learn that you teach people how to treat you and the ones that don't respect your boundaries will eventually leave, once you do start setting them. I also learned that when setting boundaries, you might have to continue to reiterate your boundaries over and over. If someone doesn't support or respect the boundaries you are putting into place, it's time to move on. If someone can't respect your boundaries, or continues to ignore the boundaries you are setting in place, they don't deserve to be in your life. This goes with friends but also family.

Another example that many of us struggle with is setting boundaries at work. When I was a teacher, setting boundaries was hard. I worked at a private school, and this one allowed parents to have our personal phone numbers. They could call whenever they wanted. They would call at all hours of the night, interrupting dinner with my family or time that was not officially my work day. One time I had a parent gift me multiple presents for my classroom and when I wouldn't do what she wanted, she demanded all of her "gifts" back. A more mature, boundary-setting version of me would have done it differently, but instead I returned all of her gifted items and spent the rest of the school year very uncomfortable. I learned the hard way that there were boundaries I needed to set. Like shutting off my phone at night and not answering calls after a certain time, not working weekends, or doing tasks outside of what my job description said. Learning to set boundaries with people teaches them what you will stand for and what you will not.

One of the hardest ways I had to learn boundary setting was becoming an entrepreneur and working from my phone. When you work from home, you spend as much time working in the pockets of time you do have all while trying to manage your other daily roles (like being a mom in my case). When you work outside of the house, you have a very set work schedule, but when you work from home, you can work all hours of the day if you aren't careful.

When I first started this life, I had absolutely no boundaries. I was working at midnight answering emails, responding to comments on my social media or sending a color match out. If my family was watching a movie, I would be over on the couch editing a video or responding to comments instead of being fully present. My job started to consume me, and I wore it like a badge of honor that I would get back to people right away and never took a day off. This behavior not only started to burn me out, but my family began feeling abandoned. Not only did I stop teaching to become more flexible with my schedule, but I wanted to be more present. Something that was not happening, due to my lack of boundaries and 24/7 service.

It took years to learn that I needed boundaries. I was so worried about hurting someone's feelings or losing out on a sale that I stopped respecting my own boundaries. After years of feeling burned out and lots of unnecessary anxiety, I decided to set official work hours for myself. I prioritized my kids and husband when they were home and worked within the pockets of my day that fit my schedule. My followers and customers easily understood and I realized it wasn't them that expected an immediate answer back—it was me. I was acting from a lacking mindset instead of an abundance mindset.

I realized that the right people would understand and the ones that didn't understand weren't for me. I learned very quickly that if someone wanted to be my customer, wanted an answer from me or needed something they would be okay to wait. I once had a lady message me on Instagram tell me she had waited 48 hours for me to email her back and she still had not heard anything. She then very rudely said maybe she should take her business elsewhere and to someone who would answer her back in 48 hours. I always respond within 24 hours so I was slightly confused. Turns out she wasn't even sending her emails to my inbox. It was a completely different email. Thankfully I had set boundaries around how I was willing to be treated by customers at this point, so I politely told her she should take her business elsewhere. I don't need customers like that in my life. Why? Because I respect my boundaries and my peace more than I do a demanding person. Thankfully I had learned by this point how I was willing to be treated by customers and have learned to let go of people like this. They are not for me.

Why is *no* such a hard word to say for so many of us? Why do we choose to do so much for others and forget that our opinions matter? This cycle of not setting boundaries that so many of us struggle with can lead to burnout and losing ourselves, our creativity, friendships and more. Our society preaches to be authentic, but when you show up "too loud" or "too much," people don't always accept you. They want you to be a little more quiet. It's like putting on a mask and pretending to be someone you aren't. The mask hides you from what you want and instead you become what other people want. You try to mold yourself to fit in. After you do that for too long, you stop knowing what you actually like or want because your decisions come from the approval of others.

How to Say NO

For so many years, I worried about disappointing others—especially my family and friends. I allowed people to walk all over me, because I was afraid if I spoke up, I would lose them. I strove for my whole life to have a good group of girlfriends. You know those commercials that show this group of tight knit friends doing everything together? Yeah, I wanted that badly. But I could never figure out why I couldn't get it. Now I realize it's because I was too busy pretending to be what others wanted me to be instead of finding real friends who thought I was perfect just the way I was. You don't need to be someone else to be accepted.

A couple of years ago, I was in a friend group of girls that I adored. I thought I had found my people, and with some of them I did. Unfortunately, things took a turn when one of the girls in the group betrayed my trust. (We'll call her Jane.) Jane was friends with another girl that was starting rumors about my daughter. This other person was creating a lot of drama in my life and hurting my child. As a mom, I knew I couldn't be around this girl or my friend Jane who was allowing it to happen. I hate confrontation and I remember sitting in Jane's car one day. I was really upset by the bullying that was happening. Jane told me to trust her and tell her what was bothering me. So, I did. I trusted that my secret would stay with her. But it didn't. She went back to the person that was bullying my daughter and told her everything I had said. The bully then messaged me and threatened me. She said the most hateful things.

I was devastated, not only because my trust had been betrayed and my friend had gossiped about me, but because this girl who

I thought was my best friend had chosen someone else. When I finally confronted Jane about it, she didn't even apologize, she just said she had to tell the bully and if I didn't like what was said, that was on me. She stuck up for the bully over me and my daughter and completely disregarded my feelings. It was like a lightbulb went off for the first time, and I realized even though I thought we were as close as sisters, she was not my friend. She didn't care about me or my family. It was that moment that my deepest fear, being abandoned became real.

We all want to feel wanted and many of us will do anything to fit in. It was in that moment, I realized I had spent years in a friend relationship wanting this girl to like me, to accept me. I was tired of being someone I wasn't. I was drained and exhausted. I hadn't set any boundaries with this relationship. This was perfectly clear when the girl didn't even seem bothered that she had hurt me. This was the moment I walked away, and after a couple of weeks of crying, I decided that I would never let myself feel or be treated that way again. I began to guard my heart and put up boundaries. I stopped allowing anyone into my life that gossiped about others and I was much more selective about who I spent my time with. I spend a lot of time self-reflecting and journaling and taking accountability for why I am a people pleaser. I also faced my fear of abandonment head on and started enjoying my own company over constantly needing others. That girl not choosing me forced me to choose myself. Today I am forever grateful for that hard time. It was a blessing that taught me more about myself and caused me to grow as a person.

It's like when we donate clothes to Goodwill, we don't look back. Why? Because we don't want them anymore. We know they will serve someone else. So why do we continually go back and check on the people in our past that don't want us? Setting boundaries helps you move on, because you begin to respect yourself too much to allow people that don't want the best for you around you.

As little girls, we are taught to be polite, to take care of others before ourselves, but keep this up and eventually you run out of energy. You are so tired from giving all your energy to others, and have none left for yourself. For so many years, I lacked the boundaries I needed to be respected and treated well. By constantly prioritizing other people's feelings, I was teaching them how to treat me when I didn't set the boundaries I needed to set. And you are too when you worry about other people's emotions over yours.

You matter. Your health matters. When you learn to set your boundaries, you may really upset some people, but the people that are upset by your boundaries are the people that don't care about you.

Trust me, the minute you start setting boundaries everything changes. As a business owner even today I still set strong boundaries. On my social media it is of utmost importance to me that I am building a community where women feel seen and heard, but I also require the same. I can't even tell you how many times I've had women come into my messages demanding something from me or asking me to change who I am.

My energy is too important to be given to difficult people. When I learned to start setting boundaries, I also saw that letting go of people that were toxic or not for me meant that I made more room for the people that deserved my time.

Life is way too short to live for others. Set the boundaries and stick with them. I promise your life will change and by respecting yourself to make these changes you will have more time to give to the life you want. Living for others and their approval will never get you to move forward in your life. Living for what you want, loving yourself and knowing your worth gives you the confidence to go after the things you desire: not what others want from you.

When you allow boundary crossers to dictate your life, your energy gets drained. When you allow people who respect your boundaries into your life, your relationships and the way you live your life change. The people you put in your life and around you play a big part in how you look at life and the perspective you have. You find respectful relationships. You don't have to change anything about yourself and you find peace because you aren't compromising parts of yourself to please others. All of a sudden you are surrounded by people who want to see you win. People who want the best for you and most of all people who respect your limits.

Bottom Line

Here's the bottom line: eliminate people in your life that want to see you fail or don't see your vision. There is no room in your life for people who drain your energy, bring you down or make you feel less-than. Lacking boundaries results in draining your energy and not following your joy. When you learn to set healthy boundaries, you are showing that your time and energy is precious. Stop thinking that setting boundaries is wrong. Instead look at boundaries as a way to start truly living the life you want and focus on spending your energy on what brings you joy, not on what drains you. You are worth it!

Here is how I started setting healthy boundaries in my life. First, I had to figure out what I was comfortable with and what I was uncomfortable with—what was I okay with allowing in my life and what did I not want. I knew that I didn't want relationships with people who gossiped about others, but I was comfortable with being around women who wanted other women to win. Knowing your limits and what drains your energy is a great way to start setting healthy boundaries. Another way I learned to set healthy boundaries was learning to practice saying no. For so many years of my life, I struggled doing this. If I didn't want to go somewhere but my friends wanted me to, I would just do it to avoid conflict. If my boss at work wanted me to put in extra hours, but I wasn't getting paid, I would do it because I didn't want to disappoint him. I realized that I was compromising my joy so that others wouldn't get mad. I started saying no when I didn't want to do something. If something was going to infringe on my time or drain my energy I just said no.

Lastly, I learned to be patient with myself. I knew that setting boundaries was something that was going to take time and lots of practice. I gave myself of grace when I would revert back to my old ways and celebrate when I was able to say no with no regrets or guilt.

Journal Questions

1. What does a healthy boundary look like for me?
2. What areas of my life do I feel my boundaries are weak?
3. What fears do I have about setting boundaries?

Makeup Mini-Tutorial: The Worst Advice I Got About Contour

What is contour, and why do you need it? Contour is ashy in color and mimics the natural shadows on the face. It can lift and recede areas of the face. This video shows you how with easy placement for more mature skin, you can get a lifted and natural sculpted look.

https://www.instagram.com/p/C4YYeI9JgrL/

Chapter Three

Fear of Failure

Think like a queen. A queen is not afraid to fail.
Failure is another stepping stone to greatness.
— Oprah Winfrey

Most people only know me as a beauty influencer, so it's surprising to find out that I was once a division one college tennis player. I started playing tennis when I was thirteen. No one in my family played tennis, but one year my parents decided they wanted a family activity, and that's what they chose. They even got books from the library to learn how to play. Not long after we started our family tennis matches, I decided to go out for the middle school tennis team.

I made it and loved it. I was a singles player and when it came time for city championships, I had no doubt in my mind that I could win. Now trust me, I had never had a lesson in my life, but I did have a crazy overachieving mindset that anything was possible, and failure was not an option.

I remember battling for that first-place spot and after hours of a close match, I came away with the trophy. The prize was a membership to our local tennis club, something we could not have afforded. My tennis journey had officially begun.

When you are starting a sport at thirteen, even back in the day, you are competing against girls who began much earlier. I honestly don't think the thought crossed my mind that I couldn't compete with them. I worked at the local clubs so that I could afford lessons and I did whatever it took to get better. Even at this young age, I would watch Wimbledon and imagine myself there. My dreams were high and so was my mindset.

Why do we lose this as we get older? When do we start doubting ourselves or telling ourselves we can't do something? When do we stop chasing our dreams simply because we are afraid of failing?

When I got to high school, I made the varsity tennis team as a freshman and continued working toward my ultimate goal: being a college tennis player. It was a hard road, and I knew it. I gave up a lot of my high school experience. Most days I would practice before and after school.

I didn't go to parties or have a lot of close friends. I honestly don't remember much about my high school experience because I was so focused on tennis, to reach a goal, sometimes you have to let go of what everyone else is doing. You have to walk your own path and I knew where I was headed.

My senior year, my doubles partner, Tara, and I competed in the state championships. We were not expected to win. Tara taught me a lot about grit. She was someone who never gave up and like me, when she wanted something she went after it. I still remember that final match to take State. She made me dig deep. I was tired, but I didn't quit. We battled and won in a close match.

After winning State, I still did not have any college tennis scholarship offers, so my tennis coach took me on a road trip to an Idaho college. He set up an appointment with the coach and we took a VHS tape of me practicing and some matches. I remember feeling I was way out of my league, but I walked up to the coach and handed him the VHS tape and listened while he talked about his program. Remember that term grit? This eighteen-year-old girl had it.

This is what I did with that college coach: I acted confident, even when I felt like the world was telling me I wasn't supposed to be there. I knew that I had what it took. The coach ended up calling me later that night and offered me a full ride Division I tennis scholarship. I was going to be a college athlete, just like I had envisioned for myself.

Let's stop here for a minute though. At any moment in time, the fear of failure could have crept in, but it didn't. It didn't because I kept myself in the moment. I took baby steps and I didn't look into the future. I didn't look at what could have gone wrong, or what could happen. I kept my eyes on what I wanted and I knew that no matter what I could reach that goal and I never doubted myself.

We all need that inner childlike confidence as we age. Maybe we need to go back to the younger version of ourselves and remember that fearlessness. As we age, we stop believing in ourselves. We are scared to try new things because we don't want to look silly or have people judge us. Here's the thing though: those people doubting you or judging you aren't moving the needle forward either. They're stuck. And you, my friend, do not have to be stuck.

I ended up playing three years of college tennis, and quit my final year of school. The girl that was so sure of herself showed up to college and was out of her league. Since I had begun my tennis career so late in life, I lacked the experience of the others had. My coach didn't believe in me. Instead, he told me a lot about myself that I started to believe instead. My confidence ebbed and I started worrying for my future. I began telling myself I wasn't good enough. Eventually, I began to hate who I was.

Self-Doubt Leads to True Failure

This was a really dark time in my life. It was the first time when I fully stopped believing in myself and I didn't even try to prove my worth because I didn't feel like I had any left. I felt lost, and this was a new feeling for me. Tennis was my identity, and not knowing what I was going to do next was one of the hardest moments in my life. I still remember calling my parents to tell them that I was going to quit. Even they tried to talk me out of it. Tennis was all I knew at the time but the thing that was once my identity was no longer bringing me joy like it once did. All of the relationships I had through tennis had become toxic. When I realized I had lost myself, I knew things needed to change, so I walked away. It would take me years later to understand, but I eventually learned that realizing something wasn't for me didn't mean I had failed. Sometimes the hardest thing is walking away from something you love, but you know is not right for you.

Self-doubt can stop us from pivoting or changing. We get so scared of the *what ifs*, that most of us just stay stuck where we are because we don't want to fail. We don't want to do something new because it may not work out. One of the biggest lessons I have learned in my life is that you honestly can't fail. You may not be amazing at everything you try, but there will be a lot of lessons that come with these new experiences. You will learn more about yourself and what you are capable of when you step out of your comfort zone. You will realize that you are stronger than you think. You can't fail at anything, because within the journey of trying something new you will learn new lessons. All of those lessons prepare you for when you find what you're meant to do. And when you find it, you'll be ready to tackle it head-on. You are meant to go through every experience. You are meant to go through the highs and the lows, because it helps you see what you want and don't want. Every challenge, every hardship and every great experience are all life's teachers. Challenges help you grow even more than the achievements.

For so many years, when I reflected on my college tennis experience I saw myself as a quitter. I had never quit at anything. I hated myself for so long for "giving up." Now that I am older, I know that experience made me better. It changed me and it prepared me for what I was to do in my future. It taught me that sometimes "quitting" or moving on is necessary. Pivoting is okay and sometimes unavoidable in order to find your happiness again.

As we age, our mind plagues us with thoughts of what we can't do. We believe those stories and they stop us from starting or doing something outside of what we know. The truth is you have to fail in order to succeed. You'll have to go through challenges to discover where you should truly be in your life. The more you fail, the more you grow. The more you fail, the more you learn about who you are and what you actually want. If you don't try or start, how will you know?

Here are two of my favorite questions that I ask myself before trying something that seems scary or hard:

1. What is the worst thing that can happen?
2. What is the best thing that can happen?

HOW TO OVERCOME FEAR

The reality check is you won't be amazing at everything you try, and you won't be perfect, but when you do try, you give yourself permission to get better. You start to unlearn old stories that have been holding you back and you lean into your gifts. Your gifts are unique to you. They are qualities and talents that you have to offer the world. Your gifts can even be your perspective on how you see things. It is up to you to share those gifts. You have the potential to change the lives around you by sharing your unique talents. You can't share your strengths if you don't know what they are, and you won't figure out your talents until you try new things. When you try new things and experience discomfort, you're giving yourself a chance for your hidden talents and gifts to shine through. When I started on social media, I was so shy. I was nervous to speak up or be different. It took me years to realize that my best talent was teaching, even though I had been a teacher for years. I realized I could use my teaching background to teach other women about makeup in a simple way. If I had never shown up on social media, I may never have known that my love of makeup combined with a love of teaching could help change the way women viewed themselves. I didn't realize how powerful my gifts could be in helping women recognize their own beauty. When you learn to trust yourself, you find what you were meant for. You find that we are all given unique talents and skill sets to share with others. By being brave and showing up—even when you don't quite feel confident—you give other people permission to do the same. It is a rolling effect. Sometimes the bravest girl in the room really isn't the most confident. She is just willing to show up and learn as she goes.

Here are some action steps to overcoming fears:

1. First acknowledge them!
2. Ask yourself: what's the worst/best thing that can happen?
3. Take baby steps—how will you start?
4. Stay in the moment. Don't move to what could happen in the future or the *what-ifs*.
5. Put yourself in new, uncomfortable situations, like starting a new hobby you've always wanted to try.

Learn to lean into what you fear and get out of your comfort zone. This is where growth happens. I was scared to leave college tennis and drop the identity I had carried for so long.

What would people think of me? I let fear win until I knew in my gut that I had to walk away. That dream wasn't meant for me anymore. I know now I hadn't failed; I had learned. And in that, I succeeded. When I finally left, a whole world opened up and I found so many other things I was good at. Likewise, you don't have to stay stuck in something because that's how people see you. You can always start over. You can always redefine yourself, but it starts with letting go of fear. When you let go of that fear of failing, you start leaning into the you that you were meant to be.

You Just Have to Start

Starting is the hardest part of doing anything. We are so afraid to go after something new because we may not be good at it. But how will we ever know what we can do if we don't try?

When I left my teaching job at 40-years-old, it was the only thing I knew. Teaching and being a mom were what I was good at, but there still felt like there was something missing. When I started showing up online, I didn't know what I was doing. I didn't know how to make a video. I didn't know how to build a business and I definitely didn't know how to teach makeup. I learned, though, and you can too. When you want something enough—when you want to change your life enough, you can figure it out. I can't tell you the countless hours I have put into learning my business. The hours I've spent watching YouTube to figure out how to do something, and asking others for help when I didn't have the skill set and learning how to fail. By failing, I mean not always getting the results I wanted. I have learned that trying new things and having them not go as planned sometimes made me feel like I was failing but in reality, I was learning what worked and what didn't work for me.

You Are Not in Competition with Anyone

You are never going to be the best at everything, and that's okay! You have a set of talents and skills that will get you exactly where you want to go. It doesn't matter if someone does it "better" than you. In my job, I've often felt like there are so many people that do it better than me. They have nicer equipment, studio lighting, and are professionally trained. But I realized that teaching is my strength and even though teaching may be someone else's strength too, they may teach in a different style than I do. That's okay, because our teaching styles speak to different people. There is room for both of us to succeed. The way you use your strengths is what makes you unique.

The fact is that there will always be someone who is better than you in someone else's eyes. There will always be someone doing it differently. You have to pave your own path and find what works for you. There will be times that you feel stuck. There will be times you will feel you aren't growing or moving fast enough. Your journey may not be as fast as someone else, but it's just right for you. There have been so many times in my journey on social media, where I have felt stuck. I wasn't seeing new followers come in. I didn't feel like my content was reaching the right people. I have felt frustrated and have wanted to give up so many times. In these moments, I reminded myself that the pace I am going is the pace I am supposed to be on.

Not Giving Up

The only "race" to win, the only "competition" you may have is you. Oftentimes we want to compare our journey to what others are doing and then we try to compare our own journey with where someone else is in theirs. Many times when you focus on what others are doing you lose focus on what you are doing. You start comparing what someone else is doing versus staying in your own lane and focusing on the process. Nothing comes quickly. Remember: This is a marathon, not a sprint. I always remind myself that I am on the exact path I am supposed to be on. And you are too! Don't worry about what Sandra down the block is doing. All of your current trials are preparing you for the greatness you were made for.

So many times, we give up when times get hard. We want to walk away and say, "This isn't meant for me" just because it gets tough. (This is different from walking away from something that is truly not meant for you.) You will never see your potential if you don't keep going.

Two years ago, if you had looked at me and my business from the outside, you would think that I was thriving. But in reality, I was a mess. *Good Morning America* had just filmed a segment on me and my Instagram account had grown to over 150k followers, but inside I was doubting myself. I felt like I was failing. My business was taking off and at a time I should have been at a high, I felt completely unsure. I had hundreds of color matches coming in from women wanting to try the makeup I was using. I had so many emails and social media messages that it took me days to respond to everyone. I started to question what I was doing, whether I could do all of it myself. Imposter syndrome was setting in. I didn't know business, but I knew I could learn. I had wanted my account to grow for so long, but when it actually happened I didn't feel prepared. What I realized was you never feel prepared. It took time for me to start trusting in myself and realizing I just needed a plan. I ended up hiring some people who could guide me in my business and help me continue to grow. I learned a lot about myself and also how to ask for help during this time. Growth can be challenging and can really push you in uncomfortable ways.

Even when you get what you want, nothing prepares you for what your thoughts tell you. My brain still told me I wasn't enough. I wasn't getting enough likes. I wasn't good enough at makeup. I wasn't pretty enough. I was too old. Our thoughts can sabotage us along the way.

The world teaches us we aren't good enough. It teaches us that we may fail, and when we start finding success it is so easy to lose ourselves and fall back on self-doubt. You will have doubt along the journey. This is normal. You have to go through tough times to see your true potential, and sometimes the uncomfortable can push you to see your greatness.

So, how do we get over doubting ourselves? How do we wade through all the stories we have been told about ourselves or the stories we have come to believe? How do we start to see our potential?

It's honestly a really easy answer. Nothing you do is about you. When we focus solely on ourselves, everything becomes about ourselves. Our problems become bigger, our messes become greater and our stories become more ingrained into our patterns.

You are a combination of your past experiences and who you are now. Your past experiences have molded you into who you are now. Your thought patterns stem from them as well. So if you want to see yourself as "good enough" you have to stop telling yourself the same old stories over and over: you have to break that pattern.

You do this by focusing on serving others, starting with your younger self. Tell your stories—without leaving out the hard details—and you start talking to that girl you once were. The more you do that, the more you will see the beauty in the messiness of life. Through this, you'll help others see that they are enough. Your experience may have made you who you are today, but they are not going to determine who you want to become. You've already "made it," because you are exactly where you are supposed to be in this moment.

Taking pride in how far you've come means you first have to wade through the mess to get there. You have to look at your past "failures" and see them instead as steps to who you are becoming.

Without your setbacks, who would you be now? Think about the times that you would consider your biggest failures. What lessons did they teach you? What did you learn from them? Did going through these "failures" improve your life or help you grow as a person? I challenge you to take time to really write these out. Look at what lessons you learned from them and then be grateful that you went through them.

Once you start telling your story, the good and the bad, you begin to feel really damn proud of yourself. You'll realize you've been through some really hard stuff, and since you made it through, you can overcome whatever life throws at you. . .because life will throw you curveballs. You will continue to doubt what you are doing at times, but you will be able to accept that feeling and move on faster instead of staying stuck in the self-doubt. That self-reflection you have done will come in helpful, because now you know who you are.

You are meant for greatness. Now is the time to accept that. Once you see yourself as who you want to be, your life will turn on its head. When your mindset changes, everything around you changes. The habits you do every day change, your attitude toward yourself and what you are doing changes and you start living the life you were meant for. Everything will change for you when you decide to start seeing yourself differently. Your words are powerful, so speak kindly and positively to yourself. Visualize the you that you want to be and start living it even if you aren't there yet.

Once I realized that I didn't have to be what others wanted me to be, I gave myself freedom to show up as myself. *That* is who people were attracted to. I could teach in a way that others couldn't. My superpower was teaching and it was helping women to see their beauty. It was helping others to feel seen. My story was unique to me, and I could share it to help others feel seen and less alone. I was meant for greatness, but so was everyone else around me. It wasn't a competition to be better or enough, I was already there, and so are you. You just have to see it. You have to recognize your greatness and once you do, you will start showing differently. We all have something in us that no one else does. Your superpower is that you are you.

When I was at the peak of the "beginning" of my career online and my account grew over 150,000 followers overnight, I was surrounded by people who believed in me. My husband, who is my biggest cheerleader, would even put post it notes around the house to remind me who I was. I would wake up to notes on our bathroom mirror reminding me of how brave I was and I still didn't believe it. I would say I believed it, but deep down I didn't. I still doubted myself. I had to work through why I was feeling this way. I had trained myself to remember why I was showing up every day. Who was I serving? I had to remember who I was; no one could do it for me. Surrounding yourself with people who believe in you, can definitely help. Putting people in your corner who cheer you on and root for you when you stop believing in yourself is critical. A strong mindset will get you far. Even when others believe in you though, you have to believe in your own self first. You have to do the inner work.

Put in the work and one day you will look in the mirror and actually see yourself and what you have to offer. The real reward comes when you can look at yourself and truly love who you are. This is when you can appreciate the journey of how far you have come and celebrate it all. You, my friend, are enough. You always were, you just had to remember it.

Journal Questions:

1. What fears are holding you back from what you really want?
2. What is one baby step you could do today to start to overcome your fear?
3. How do you feel when you let fear control your decisions?

_____

_____

_____

_____

_____

_____

_____

_____

_____

_____

_____

_____

_____

_____

_____

_____

_____

_____

_____

_____

Makeup Mini-Tutorial: Concealer Hack for Over 40

The biggest thing most of us notice as we age? Fine lines and wrinkles under the eyes. As we age, we hold more texture under the eyes and applying more product there can just accentuate it. Here are my tricks for getting the perfect undereye!

https://www.instagram.com/p/C3VlzzyPygf/

Chapter Four

Blessings in Disguise

You gain courage, strength and confidence by every experience that you stop and look fear in the face. You can say to yourself, I lived through this trauma, I can take the next thing that comes along.

— Eleanor Roosevelt

A note before you continue: This chapter discusses birth trauma and experiences with NICU babies, which may be emotionally challenging for some readers. Please proceed with care."

I became pregnant with my first baby when I was 26 years old. I was still teaching at the time and my husband had almost graduated from Physician Assistant school. As you can imagine, we were so excited to start our little family and become parents. We did all the routine doctor's visits—all firsts for us and our baby boy looked so strong and healthy. As we got closer to his due date, we had everything ready for his arrival. His room was ready and set up and we started counting down the date to his arrival. As it got closer, the doctors realized he was breech, and because I didn't want a C-section, they decided to try and turn him in utero. Luckily, that went well and he turned head-down. But because they were worried, he wouldn't stay that way, they decided to deliver him a week early.

We arrived at the hospital the morning of my induction nervous, but excited to finally meet our son. We had no clue what we were doing, but we were sure ready to be parents. Jackson James finally arrived on April 24, 2007 after fifteen hours of labor and weighed a whopping six pounds and five ounces. He didn't cry at first, and I remember them rubbing his body until he did. He was perfect.

We stayed in the hospital for a full day and Jackson had a pretty hard time latching to feed and the lactation nurse spent a lot of time with us helping us. When it was time to leave the hospital and go home, we promised to bring him back in a couple of days and report his feeding progress.

Two days after we went home with our newborn, our world forever changed. I still remember vividly getting that call from the lactation nurse asking how Jax was doing. I reported back that he seemed kind of weak and really struggled with feeding. The nurse suggested we bring him in and I told her I didn't think it was urgent.

You know those moments in life, when the universe or God or whatever you believe in, gives you a sign? I remember putting the phone down and locking eyes with my husband. At the same time, we both said, "Let's just bring him in."

As we drove to the hospital, Jackson was extremely quiet and seemed so tired. We didn't know any better. We were new parents and thought that he just slept a lot. When we got to the hospital, we took him out of the car seat and he was breathing really rapidly and strangely. He was blue. The doctors immediately took him from us and put him in an oxygen tube. He was struggling to breath and was sitting at 60% oxygen.

We didn't understand. We didn't know what was wrong, but even though the nurses and doctors were trying to stay calm the busyness of what was going on signaled otherwise. They ushered us into a room without our baby and told us something was wrong with Jackson's heart. They had already sent him to be flown out to Primary Children's Hospital in Utah, which was over three hours away from us. They told us to pack our bags and drive there to meet him. They didn't know if he would make it.

I wish I could describe my exact feelings in that moment. The sheer panic. The thoughts that went through my mind. The lack of understanding what was happening around me. The look of fear across my husband's face, who medically knew more than me...but I can't. It seems like such a blur.

Sometimes in life, you get thrown some major curveballs. You get given things you didn't ask for. Things that don't seem fair. Somehow though, your body just moves even when you feel frozen and you get through it. You don't have time to feel the feelings, you just do it. The hurried packing of our bags before driving three hours to the hospital, hoping our baby would be alive when we arrived. The drive to Utah, shaking and scared but just putting one foot in front of the other to get there. The adrenaline that comes with trauma.

When we arrived at the hospital, our baby was on so many drugs. His kidney function and blood flow from his chest down was shut down and he was attached to wires and tubes and there were doctors and nurses surrounding him trying to keep him stable. We had no clue what the next month and a half would have in store for our lives and our baby.

We later found out that Jackson was born with an interrupted aortic arch, meaning that candy cane shaped tube that was supposed to move blood from his heart to the rest of his body didn't exist. He also had two large holes in his Atrial Septal Defect and his Ventricular Septal Defect. We learned our two-day-old baby would have open heart surgery in order to stay alive.

I began to question my faith during this time. I spent every day at that hospital, pumping in a hospital bathroom, singing to my boy, telling him he was strong and resilient, all while questioning why this was happening to us. I would sit in the hospital garden crying and asking God why, and not getting an answer.

Jackson had his surgery and thanks to the amazing staff at Primary Children's Hospital, he is now seventeen years old and a senior in high school. He has had some challenges with his heart, but has healed amazingly. To say he is our miracle is an understatement. He has taught me to believe in miracles. He has taught me to believe that we are all here for a greater purpose, and he has taught me that life is precious.

We all have hard things happen to us. This experience taught me that you never know what someone is going through. Most people will have something hard happen at one point in their lives. Going through something like this taught me perspective. I spent a lot of years wrestling with why this happened to our family—why we had to go through this with our baby. I was so angry because this was not at all how I imagined my life. I later realized after working through so many emotions, that how we choose to look at the hard, determines how we live life and how we take advantage of the life we have. I met so many mamas in that heart unit that lost their babies or were told their babies also had congenital heart defects and I wish I had an answer. It's unfair. The hard things that happen, even though we don't understand them, have the ability to wake us up. They teach us to truly live life, because it's short. We only have this small time on Earth to make an impact, so why aren't we doing it?

Many people ask me how we handled everything as we navigated Jackson and his healing. It was the hardest thing I have ever gone through. Years later, and many hours of dealing with the way this trauma affected me and my family, I came to understand that life can be taken from you at any minute. As hard as it was for many years to tell this story, I realized that telling your story can change lives and help others feel less alone. A story that changes the way others look at their lives as well can be really powerful too. I also learned from this experience how you can never judge someone else's story. You never know what someone is going through. You never know what trauma they have lived and I think it teaches us to have some compassion when dealing with others.

Hard Things I've Learned

Almost losing my baby was one of the most challenging experiences I've ever gone through. I learned that life isn't always roses and sunshine and that hard times are going to happen in life, and it will likely hurt. Those hard times help us to find out how much strength we actually have in us. This lesson was one I wouldn't learn until years after Jackson's surgery. It took a lot of processing and accepting to be able to see the blessings that came from Jackson and our family going through this. It is still scary and it is still something I of course wish had never happened. There have been times where this condition has affected how Jackson lives his life and there have been many moments where I can't stop crying and worrying about him. Jackson has been so resilient and calm through all of this. He has taught me how important it is to not only stay in the moment instead of worrying about the future, but also how fast life can be taken from us. We have found so much strength from watching Jackson navigate the life he has been given. It has taught us to not take anything or anyone for granted.

Sometimes we have to be at our lowest point to find our strength again and that timeline looks different for everyone. Going through really hard things, like losing someone you love, or watching them feel pain so great that you question your faith and existence. I know I did. I went through a lot of emotions. I was mad. Mad at God for giving my son this issue he would have for the rest of his life. I was mad that this was my first experience as a mom. I was also sad: sad watching my little boy in so much pain at just a week old. I felt scared. How was this going to affect my son for the rest of his life? How was I going to protect him? Sometimes in life the hard things make us question what really matters.

Do you ever stop and look around at the life you are creating? Do you ever question whether this is what you want? The hard lessons in life can either break you or mold you. How you decide to write your next steps is up to you. It's ok to feel the feelings— to cry, to want to give up. To acknowledge the hard. Sometimes it's the baby steps you do each day that heal you, that show you the gratitude in the situation.

Going through this hard time made our family closer; my relationship with my husband changed for the better. Watching my son grow in his resilience and drive to accomplish his dream regardless of his trauma has shaped us all. You may not see the underlying blessings in the hard right away, but one day you will. Hard things shape us, they change us and they are part of our journey in finding ourselves again.

Tough Times Growing Up

When I was just five years old, my family went through a time that molded me into how I chose to look at life. Despite my young age, watching how my parents embraced and accepted difficult situations has stuck with me until this very day.

In 1986, there was an oil price collapse. My family lived in San Antonio, Texas at the time. My dad was making a great income as a Landscape Architect in a firm that was well known, so we were easily able to afford two homes and multiple expensive cars. But when the oil crisis happened, there was a big recession and my dad suddenly lost his job.

My mom was a teacher and didn't know how she would go back to work with two small kids and be able to afford the prices that came with childcare in a bigger city. My parents decided to move to a small town called Marshall, TX. Looking back, I am sure that was not an easy decision. My dad decided to work in the ministry as a teacher at the local church school. My mom took to babysitting other church members' children during the day to make extra money.

We rented a small, older house with a carport. I still remember spending hours roller-skating under that carport. We had one car for my dad to get to work, but it needed a lot of electrical fixes that we couldn't afford, so to get into the car, I had to crawl through the windows because the door wouldn't work. My dad also took a part time job selling suits and ties at the local Dillard's for extra money and even then, many of our clothes were bought at garage sales.

We also lived in a lower income neighborhood. One day, I was playing with my brother when our ball went over our neighbor's fence. We hopped the fence to search for it, and as we were looking through the weeds we found a hypodermic needle. I remember my mom's face when I told her what we found. We were gaining experiences at an early age that she wasn't comfortable with.

My parents knew we had to get out of that house, so we moved into a bigger house and shared it with a fellow church member. I was only about eight years old and I will never forget this house. It was old with the biggest porch I had ever seen, complete with a porch swing that we would swing on for hours. There was so much land. I can remember spending my days, after being homeschooled, looking for roly polys, making elaborate bike tracks with my brother out of old bricks we found in the garage, and exploring the land around us. My mom made homemade tortillas and we ate a lot of beans and rice, because it was cheap. Looking back I know my parents didn't have much money, but I felt like the happiest kid in the world.

A year and a half later, my parents decided that we needed to move and start a different life. My mom found a National Geographic magazine and inside she saw an article on a place called Boise. It was the capital city of Idaho and the mountains intrigued her. My dad decided to take a trip out west with a friend, and when he was out there, he happened to get two different job offers in Boise. So with a truckload of belongings and a whole lot of faith, we packed up and moved.

Even though I was little, these experiences shaped me. From the outside looking in, you could totally say we were poor and had nothing. In my eyes, we had everything. My parents taught me to always have gratitude during the hard times as much as the great ones. I learned a lot during this time and discovered that material things don't matter. What matters most are the moments we have and how important family is. The hard moments teach us a lot about ourselves. There is a reason we go through it all, even if we don't quite understand it then. I learned that material things don't matter—family matters. The people around you matter. The material things can disappear at any moment, but those relationships and lessons you learn while you are wading through the not-so-great things never leave you.

Learning to Look Through a Lens of Gratitude

How did I learn to look at every hard experience with gratitude? I changed my lens. I asked myself what is this situation supposed to be teaching me. What am I supposed to be learning? Even though the answers weren't clear for several years, I knew they would always come.

I had faith that no matter what is happening, this was the best possible thing that could be happening in that moment. When you realize that life is always happening *for* you and not *to* you it changes your perspective. Life is here to teach us, to help us grow and to help us find grace in every moment.

Everything that happens to you is supposed to happen. That's why when we compare our lives to someone else's, we may feel sad or even depressed. Your life is teaching you what you need to learn. The person you're watching through your phone screen is on their own path and struggling in ways you probably can't see.

The people that walk into our lives are all teachers. They are all meant to teach us more about who we want to be. They are teaching us to learn to let go. That broken marriage, the relationship that didn't work out...you needed to go through it so you have more clarity on what you want and what you deserve. Maybe you're meant to pick up the pieces of that relationship down the road, but first you need to learn more about yourself. By finding gratitude in every situation, you allow yourself to grow and heal. Every situation and person are meant to teach us a lesson, it is our job to find it. There are so many blessings all around us; sometimes we just have to stop and find what life is truly teaching us. Blessings are situations, good or bad, that are meant to teach you about yourself, change your life trajectory or put you on a path that has a better outcome. Sometimes when we don't understand why a situation is happening to us, it can take years later to actually see the blessing in it.

Once you understand that every situation and person is a teacher, you start learning how to navigate the challenging times with new glasses. When I quit my job as kindergarten teacher, my social media didn't just take off. I spent more hours than I can count working, being away from my family, self-doubt and pivoting in the wrong direction. But the thing is, "wrong" direction wasn't wrong. I needed to go through it to get to where I am today.

When I started on social media, I honestly didn't know what I was doing. I knew I was talking to women about makeup, but I didn't truly know yet what my purpose was. I dabbled in talking about my teens and the funny things they did. I talked about being a mom and I worked through a lot of what I was struggling with online. I told stories of lost friends and how to gain confidence and I used all of this time to learn who I was talking to. I didn't gain followers right away, but I did start to find myself and gain an understanding of who I was and what I wanted to be. Along the way, I started figuring out who I was talking to, what my mission was, and who I was trying to serve and then my followers began to grow. I was building a community of women who were going through similar life situations and felt less alone.

So when you look at someone, when you go to judge someone else's life or decision, remember this...they are going through exactly what they need to be going through in that moment.

Treating people with compassion and giving others grace is so important, because we have never walked in their shoes. Everyone's path is different. Everyone's story is different, and if we didn't have our "hard" we couldn't tell our story and help others feel that they can make it through their "hard" too. Sharing your story, even though it is uncomfortable, can help others feel less alone. Sharing our stories not only helps us as we navigate them, but it helps others realize that they aren't alone in what they are going through.

Journal Questions

1. What past experiences, especially challenging ones, are you grateful for and how have they shaped you? What blessings can you find in the hard and challenging experiences?
2. Who is around you that you are grateful for? Who cheers you on, even when you don't cheer yourself on? Find people in your circle that lift you up and are key players when you are going through challenging situations.
3. How can you find gratitude in the boring or routine aspects of your life? Finding gratitude even in the mundane everyday tasks helps you experience gratitude in your life. Sometimes we get bored with our simple lives, but there are so many blessings every day!

_____

_____

_____

_____

_____

_____

_____

_____

_____

_____

_____

_____

_____

Makeup Mini-Tutorial: Perimenopause Stole My Joy at 42

My road to learning I was in perimenopause was a long one. In fact, I am sure I had more symptoms earlier, but I just didn't listen to my body. Here is a story of how I lost my joy, but found it again—and how you can too!

https://www.instagram.com/p/C5CdOH0uW1d/

Chapter Five

Getting out of your comfort zone

Do one thing every day that scares you.
— Eleanor Roosevelt.

I remember the first videos I made for social media. I didn't know what I was doing. I was 39 years old, super shy and deathly scared of what people would think of me. I was using filters to hide my "flawed" skin because every influencer I saw had beautiful perfect skin. I remember the first time I went live on Facebook. It was something I had never done before. I still remember nervously pushing the record button and hoping I could get through it without throwing up.

I pushed record and shakily held up my makeup and said a couple of words; to this day I don't even remember what I said because everything seemed jumbled up in my head. I started talking and as I was applying my makeup, my hand hit the pile of books stacked up high on the chair holding a tiny ring light and my phone (I didn't even know what a ring light was at the time) and the entire setup fell to the ground and toppled over— all while I was still LIVE.

I remember panicking and quickly picking up the pile of books and the ring light and the phone and saying to the two people on my live (which felt like a lot at the time) that if they wanted to see awkward they had come to the right place. I laughed and to this day, I live my business this way. Authenticity will always win. I show up now without filters. I show up on social media when I am happy, when I am sad, when I am having a hard day. I show up because I want women to see that real life isn't perfect. We have emotions, sometimes we feel bloated, and we have days where someone said something so mean it made us want to crawl into a hole and never come out again. This is normal and okay. I have learned to show up unapologetically and authentically me and the right people will stick around. I don't pretend to be someone I am not anymore.

You are never going to be perfect. You are never going to always know what you are doing, but you just have to start. You have to start even when you don't feel confident. You have to start when you don't feel good enough. You have to start without having knowledge. You just have to show up and do it every day. That's how you learn to get out of your comfort zone.

If I had a dollar for every comment on social media that attacked my looks or my intentions, I would be rich. People are always going to judge. They are always going to assume. I have had people be triggered just by me showing up as myself. They don't like my body, the moles on my face, my age spots, and the list could go on. For a long time, I didn't understand why, but as I have gained confidence I realized that people's reactions toward me have nothing to do with me. It has everything to do with their own insecurities. It has everything to do with them, not me. When you show up happy, people will always try to dim your light.

You may be scared to start a new hobby, change a career, or jump into that relationship, but how will you know if you don't even try?

There have been so many times in my career on social media that I haven't felt comfortable. There have been times I didn't know what I was doing, but if I hadn't had the guts to try, I wouldn't be where I am today. Listen, you are going to fail. You aren't going to be good right away and you definitely won't always know what you are doing.

Most people look at your life as a highlight reel—they don't know what you have been through. My son's open-heart surgery, struggling to find my identity after quitting tennis, learning to let go of people who weren't for me and watching my family go through hard times were all experiences that have shaped me and prepared me. They have taught me how to accept what life has dealt me and it has helped me better relate to others.

These tough life trials or hardships are preparing you for where you are going to be someday. The hard times, what might seem like setbacks can be frustrating. Trust me, I have spent many hours crying and upset when something I thought should have worked out and didn't, only to realize it was in my best interest. It took me years to realize that my best friend gossiping about me and choosing another person over me was something I needed to go through to learn what real friendships were and how to set boundaries.

Over the years, I've learned to have gratitude for the journey, because it's all a part of reaching my goals. If everything was easy, we wouldn't appreciate it. Think about situations where you have gotten what you wanted right away. I bet they aren't as easy to recall as something that took you longer to get, but when you did you felt so proud of yourself. Sometimes looking back from where you started to where you are now is the best remedy when you think you aren't achieving your goals. Pushing yourself to live out of your comfort zone teaches you that you can do hard things. Pushing yourself out of your comfort zone proves you're capable of doing hard things. And those hard things? They're the very challenges that lead to growth and transformation.

From teaching makeup classes to women, appearing on podcasts, being on *Good Morning America*, and even writing this book...I've been scared. I am not a natural speaker. I am not someone who wants to be in front of a room full of people; in fact, I'm the girl who turns beat red when I have to speak to a crowd. But I'm also not the girl to say no to a challenge. I truly believe that anyone can figure out something if they want it bad enough. Getting out of your comfort zone and trying something new takes time. For years, I had to work hard at showing up online even when I was uncomfortable or didn't want to. I didn't see fast results, but I did find that the more I worked on myself, the more I started to not feel as uncomfortable. I did this through journaling, working on my mindset and putting positive people around me. The more I practiced and worked on me, the more I actually started to feel more confident in who I was and where I was going.

You know the story of the tortoise and the hare? It's the same principle for when you decide to do something new. The fastest person out of the gate doesn't win the race. The winner is the person who is consistent. The one who doesn't give up. The woman who works intentionally and slowly toward her goal will eventually see the reward. In our world, everyone wants results fast, and when they don't get what they want right away, most people quit. I'm here to tell you that nothing comes fast, because if it did you wouldn't appreciate the tears, time and effort it took to reach what you wanted. All the trials and hardships made you this new person. They taught you new skills that you will need when you finally get to where you want to be.

Getting out of your comfort zone is a journey. It doesn't happen overnight. It's a road of self-discovery. It starts with first recognizing that you are uncomfortable. The next steps are the hardest because they are the ones where you have to dig deep to find out where the uncomfortable is stemming from. Is it from our childhood? Have you had experiences in your past where others have taught you that you aren't enough? Maybe you have been told you weren't good at something and subconsciously, you believed it. All of these thoughts and ingrained feelings we have are holding us back from being who we really are. We believe from an early age the things others have told us and so unlearning them takes time. The unlearning part can be really uncomfortable, because for many of us it takes questioning your beliefs and the deep rooted thoughts we have had about ourselves for so long.

It's not a destination—it doesn't take trying one time to "get it." You are changing repeated thought patterns and behaviors.

This takes a lot of self-reflection and time (and yes, maybe even some therapy). You don't need to be the first person to cross the finish line, because it's not even a race. It sometimes takes those baby steps to get a little confidence to take the next step. The more steps you take, you may start looking back and realize you are doing it! You are doing the things that scare you!

When I started showing makeup tips on social media, no one was watching. I maybe got a few likes on a post and it seemed like I wasn't making a difference. I felt like no one was noticing me. It was hard. I realized early on that I had to believe in myself first before anyone would believe in me. There were times I wanted to quit. Instead, I started doing my research. What were the pain points my age group was experiencing with makeup and how could I help? I started sharing tiny tips to make makeup easy, and guess what? People began watching and trying them. Soon, messages poured into my inbox saying my tips were working, and their confidence was beginning to grow. When I focused less on how stupid I felt and more on how I could help others, my comfort zone became more comfortable.

No One Cares, Troll

Getting out of your comfort zone requires you to let go of what others think of you. But when you do things based on the opinions of others, you're letting them determine your future. Maybe you wanted to be an astronaut but you were told that could never happen. If you spend a large amount on a car, someone is going to have an opinion. If you change your hair, someone won't like it. Your great aunt will ask you why you haven't lost your baby weight, but when you do drop those extra pounds your grandma will tell you you're too skinny. If you hear this enough times, eventually you start believing in what someone else's opinion of you is, and you start believing it too. Letting go of the weight of other people's opinions is incredibly liberating. The main reason other people judge you is because they're too scared of going after what they want. Instead of putting in the work themselves, they're busy judging you from the sidelines.

You don't want people like that in your corner. Remember the boundaries I talked about in earlier chapters? You will need these. Your true friends will lift you up—the people who don't want the best for you will not. They will say things to dim your light and they will not support you along the way. Stop believing the things that people tell you that you are. What you believe about yourself is what matters. Self-reflecting, focusing on your mindset, and showing up, unapologetically will move you closer to your goals. At the end of the day when you look in the mirror, the only opinion that matters is yours. The things people say to you have no weight. I hope that you can look at yourself and be proud of who you are becoming.

Someone once told me that when I started getting trolls online, I had made it. Listen, friend, if you have lofty goals, then you better believe there will be people rooting against you. It's ok if people don't like you, if they don't get you. You aren't for everyone. Follow your own path, it will look different from someone else's. Mute the haters in your life and at the end of the day be proud of who you are and what your goals are.

The more emotional energy you give to other people, the more unfocused you become toward your own goals. If you want to make an impact on the world, stop taking what other people think of you personally. As Don Miguel Ruiz says in his book *The Four Agreements*, "Nothing other people do is because of you. It is because of themselves." What he means is, whatever happens around you, don't take anything personally.

For so many years, I was so stuck in playing it safe. I didn't want to ruffle feathers. I was scared to try things that made me nervous. Until one day, I looked around at my three small kids and realized I was showing them how to do the same. From that day on, I made it a goal to do things that made me nervous. I was scared of water, so we took a day trip to go cliff jumping. I was afraid of heights, so I booked us a trip to walk on the glass floor of the space needle. The more I proved to myself that I could do things that scared me, the less scared I was to try more new things. It was like a domino effect.

Doing hard things forces you into discomfort. Living in the uncomfortable and the messy helps you grow into a stronger person who doesn't let fear run their life. Your next step, again, is to just start. You never know where life can take you once you begin putting yourself into spaces you never thought you could fit into. In fact, you might be surprised at where life will take you.

Journal Questions:

1. What holds you back from doing what you want to do?
2. What past experiences have shown you that stepping out of your comfort zone can help you?
3. What are some things you could do to step out of your comfort zone?

_____

_____

_____

_____

_____

_____

_____

_____

_____

_____

_____

_____

_____

_____

_____

_____

_____

_____

_____

_____

_____

Makeup Mini-Tutorial: How to Place Eyeshadow as We Age

As we age, our eyes are one of the first areas visibly affected. If you didn't have hooded eyes from birth, you may notice that the lid space of your eye has gotten smaller. This is totally normal and this video will show you an easy strategy to get your eye looking more lifted and youthful.

https://www.instagram.com/p/C1XYNNrOzhX/

Chapter Six

Be Authentic

Authenticity is about the choice to show and be REAL. The choice to be HONEST. The choice to let our true selves be seen.

— Brené Brown

I spent so much of my life trying to fit in. I wanted so badly to be the girl that everyone liked, but for some reason I could never be that girl. I always felt different. When I was in fourth grade, my family moved to Boise, Idaho and I was the new girl in a school where everyone knew each other. I felt like the outsider. My first memory of that classroom was the day I mustered enough courage to speak in class.

Back in my home state of Texas, we were taught southern manners and that included addressing every adult as "Sir" or "Ma'am." When we answered a question in class, we would stand next to our desk and precede our response with a "Yes ma'am."

Well, when I decided to finally speak up in my new Idaho class, this shy fourth grade kid stood up next to her chair to answer and everyone started to snicker. The heat crept up from my neck into my face and I quickly sat down. This was the first time I remember feeling like I needed to sit down and be quiet because I was different and like I "stuck out." After a while, it was easier to stay quiet and not be noticed.

I think so many of us have felt this way, whether you were that shy kid who secretly wanted to be a part of the popular group or the girl who looked like she had a lot of friends, but those "friends" constantly left her out or talked about her behind her back. As women, we are taught to be quiet, fit in and not stand out from a young age.

I look at my fifteen-year-old daughter as she navigates her high school year. She is way more confident than I ever was. I do see her worry about what to wear, and who posts what on social media. Normal things, but also important to communicate about. Their brains are still so underdeveloped, so it is easy to conform or follow trends just because they are seeing it online. The way that she is living her high school years is much different than I did. I try to monitor what she sees on social media, and we talk a lot about choosing the right friends that accept her for who she is. Seeing the pressures from social media gives me even more reason to preach the authenticity message.

We are so inundated with messages all around us telling us as women, to play small and change who we are. Growing up, we watched tv shows and commercials telling women they needed to lose weight, or to buy a certain skincare routine to be beautiful, or even to smoke cigarettes to look sexy. As a young girl, I judged my body harshly in the mirror, questioning my looks—whether my pores were small enough and waist the correct size. Now that I have a daughter, I think about the young girl I was and I never want her to feel that way about herself.

As I got older, I was never the girl surrounded by a lot of friends. I wanted so desperately to have close girlfriends that I could confide in but I struggled to find loyal girlfriends. I spent so many of my years trying to fit into the "cool girl group," but these girls would leave me out, talk behind my back or pretend I wasn't there.

I don't think enough people talk about what it's like to not have a lot of girlfriends. Social media shows a world where everyone is happy and has friends. These girls are always out on a girl's vacay wearing matching pajamas, dressed and laughing together at a party, or drinking wine and eating pizza at their own "Friendsgiving" or "Galentine's Day."

In my early adult years, I made friends with girls who seemed to be so cool. I found myself dressing like them, decorating my house like them, and falling into patterns that even included gossiping about others. It was exhausting. I wasn't me, but I felt that in order to have friends who liked me I had to be someone I wasn't.

Haven't we all been there at one time or another, pretending to be someone we aren't just to fit in? We are all so dang worried about being judged if we show up as ourselves that we pretend to be something we aren't. A lot of us are trying to be perfect to fit in. We pretend we have a squeaky-clean house, that we are raising the perfect kids, and even showcase an ideal marriage. I once read a quote, "Don't be perfect, be real." You know what brings people together? Realness. You know what doesn't? Being perfect. Why? Because no one is perfect. When you step outside and look honestly at your life, most of us are living a messy life and trying to just survive.

If you're like me, then you hide the struggles of your daily life because you're scared what people might think of you if they knew the truth. We are so worried about the judgment of someone we hardly know that we pretend to be who we are not. But guess what? If you actually showed up imperfect, you might start connecting with others more than you realize.

We also pretend to have a picture-perfect life, because if we actually let people in, we would have to be honest with ourselves. Our insecurities are our indicators of what we fear we are lacking. This goes back to stories we were told as kids— we have to face these if we want to find true friendship and connections.

For example, in my social media world, you have to have your hair done, makeup on, and nails perfect in order to be seen and avoid being judged. For years, I wouldn't go to the grocery store without a full face of makeup and my hair right because I didn't want other people to think I wasn't put together. I eventually realized that I learned this subconsciously from a relative who never stepped foot outside of the house without her hair perfectly coiffed and a full face of makeup. I had to decide for myself if that was a standard that I truly wanted to hold myself to (I did not). Coming to this realization wasn't immediate: it took some self-reflection to figure out why I felt I needed to look perfect for my weekly Target run.

When I hit my forties, it was like a lightbulb went off in my head. I didn't want to be like everyone else. I didn't want to just "fit in" anymore. I was tired of surrounding myself with people who were only pretending to be my friends, but when I left the room would talk shit about me. I wanted to be me, and if someone didn't like who I was then they weren't for me. Learning to set boundaries helped me so much with this. When I was clear and upfront with what I would allow in my life, the people who weren't for me suddenly disappeared. True friends accept your boundaries and allow you to be truly you.

Showing Up as Me

Showing up on social media in the beginning was really hard for me. I was so afraid to be myself to a world of strangers. I wanted followers and in order to gain them, I felt like I had to be someone I wasn't. I had to have people like me, so they would push that follow button. I didn't want to be too loud or too much and so I played it really safe. I showed up with filters to hide my older, imperfect skin. I showed up in my stories with a clean house, well dressed and always with makeup on.

I will never forget the moment one of my friends, who was also on social media, called me one day and asked me why I always show up with a filter or with a perfect face of makeup on. I remember laughing and saying, "No one wants to see me any other way." I remember this friend saying to me. "Yes, people want to see you messy. They want to relate." I thought about it for a while and then she challenged me to record my social media story the minute I got out of bed the next morning. She said, "Just do it and see what happens."

What happened next was that more people started to feel seen. More women related to me because I was showing messiness. I realized that if you want people to relate to you, then you have to be authentically you. This is contrary to everything we're taught as women: to silence our voices and hide our imperfect lives.

Since I'm from a small town, I would instinctively try to live a private life. I didn't want people to gossip about me. If you have ever lived in a smaller town, you know that everyone knows everyone and there is always history. I was worried about people talking about me. I was worried about their judgments. I was worried about their assumptions, so much so that I didn't want to show up as me.

But as I started to show myself, I felt so much freedom. I started talking about topics that I was dealing with and more women began messaging me. The more they shared their stories with me, and the less alone I felt. I realized that when you share your stories and experiences, you give others permission to share theirs too.

Showing my imperfect self actually helped me work through my traumas of being not enough. It made me feel less alone, and more women related to what I was going through too. No one has it all together. No one doesn't have a hard moment. We are all struggling with something. We have all cried in our closets at one point and hidden our disappointments. We have all felt alone, left out and not good enough. We need to share those moments. We need to normalize that life is hard, and that we can show that part of our lives. . .along with your resilience.

The last four years of being on social media, I have shown up in every way imaginable. Happy, sad, disappointed, anxious, strong, and empty. I showed up when my sweet dog died suddenly, when my best friend moved away and when we thought my seventeen-year-old son may need open heart surgery again. I showed up unshowered, upset and crying. Each time I showed up authentically, the women online who I cultivated relationships through that authenticity reached out to me to offer support, sympathy, and encouragement that helped me keep going.

I have also shown up in good times in my life. I show my day-to-day life of driving three hours one way to take my daughter to soccer practice a couple of times a week. I show how I have struggled with my perimenopause journey and also celebrated when I started feeling like myself again. I don't hold back online, because I want women to feel seen. Taking women to go get Botox with me because they are considering getting it done is just another way I continue to show up in every way of my life even if someone doesn't agree with my life choices.

I have shared my authentic self with the women who follow me in hopes that they stop for a minute and realize that their *life* is reality, not what they are seeing on their screens. I have fostered relationships with women who have needed a space to talk to someone. These relationships have improved my life and my business, and without authenticity, I would never have made them in the first place.

However, some people are going to be triggered by you being your authentic self. They think you should act a certain way, say things differently, or want you to get over things quickly if you are struggling. It took me years to tell those people that I am human. That I can process things however I want. I can respond to comments in any way I want and I will not silence my voice to be someone I'm not. I have traumas. I am human and I react in ways I am not always proud of, but at the end of the day I love myself even more for always showing up as me.

While struggling with perimenopause, I gained fifteen pounds, and I shared how I handled the weight gain and losing it again in my videos. Many women were happy I shared this part of my journey because they wanted to know how they could handle it. Others were upset. They believed I already had the ideal body type, and talking about losing the weight was problematic. I realized that what they felt had nothing to do with me — it was their insecurities and fears that were upsetting them. That doesn't mean I should stop being my authentic self.

You will always have critics in your life. But that doesn't mean you have to stop being you. I encourage you to be yourself. To look at how you respond to situations or people. Are you living an authentic life or one that reflects how the people around you want you to be? Pretending to be someone you aren't is exhausting. Dress how you want, speak up when you want, set boundaries and say no when you don't feel like doing something. It might not seem like much, but those baby steps are giant steps to living an authentic and free life.

Giving up the lies and showing up honest that's what creates the life of your dreams. Doing things for others or being someone you're not is not a life worth living. I promise, the moment you start living for you is the moment the world opens up for you.

How Do I Start Showing Up as Myself?

How I learned to show up authentically me:

1. I learned that in order to be me, I had to be in perfect alignment with my values, belief systems and who I was. I had to stop apologizing for who I was.
2. I learned to set boundaries. People got mad at me and some even stopped being my friend when I did this. You have to learn to protect your peace without compromising your values or people will always walk all over you. Learn to say no.
3. I learned to love who I am. When you learn to accept yourself and put your own needs first, authenticity happens. You put yourself in places you want to be, not places you have to be.

If you aren't sure who you want to be through the noise of others' expectations, then trust your gut. Ask yourself whether something is a hard yes or a hard no. If something is a hard no for me, I absolutely will not do it. It wasn't meant for. And if it's a hard yes. . . well then I've found one more arrow pointing me to who I truly want to be.

Journal Questions:

1. What past experiences have taught you that it is scary to be authentic or show up as yourself? Journal these experiences and start small. Ask yourself what benefits you got from the experience that you can see now that you didn't see then. If you find these experiences feel traumatic to relive, seek outside help to work through them in the most healthy way for you.
2. How would you describe yourself when you are being 100% authentically you?
3. Are there role models in your life that encourage you to show up as yourself? Write down how they encourage you.

_____

_____

_____

_____

_____

_____

_____

_____

_____

_____

_____

_____

_____

_____

_____

_____

Makeup Mini-Tutorial: Updated Black Eyeliner

Are you still wearing your eyeliner like you did in your twenties? I was guilty of it too! If you love black eyeliner, you can still wear it. This video will show you how you can still use black eyeliner but get a more updated look.

https://www.instagram.com/p/C2Yktvxp0xr/

Chapter Seven

Confidence

The most important day is the day you decide you are good enough for you, it's the day you set yourself free.

— Unknown

As I've said before, I was a driven kid who not only wanted to succeed: I wanted to be exceptional at everything I did. That drive only increased as I got older. I probably looked pretty confident, but this was a façade. I was always struggling with acceptance.

As I mentioned in chapter four, we didn't have a lot of money when I was growing up. I honestly don't remember noticing. My parents never instilled a belief in the importance of owning a lot of things. They taught me to have faith and that your worth wasn't built on physical things. My strongest memories aren't of going to school in my garage-sale wardrobe, but people around me, the memories of playing outside until my mom called us inside, and all the fun I had.

Having a childhood not focused on "things" taught me to embrace the moments.

When I reached middle and high school, I became more aware of what people were wearing and wanted to look like them too. I remember school shopping one year with my mom shopping at an old department store called Bon Marche. We had a one-hundred-dollar budget for the entire year. We would often times use layaway to keep our stuff until my parents got paid and we could go back and get them. I wanted to be like those rich girls who could have whatever they wanted, and not being able to dress like them hurt my confidence, but I still felt blessed because I knew how hard my parents worked to give me what I wanted and I learned to appreciate what I did have.

In college, I was blessed enough to have all of my school paid for thanks to tennis. I worked really hard during that time to graduate without any debt. My confidence started to dip in college however, due to some of my tennis experiences and the people I had placed in my life. I struggled a lot with my self-esteem and my weight during this time.

I noticed my confidence really started to deteriorate when I was a stay-at home-mom. My kids were 22 and 24 months apart and I felt so isolated at times because it was so much work taking three kids to go anywhere. I didn't have a lot of friends and the only people I was really around was when we would do playdates. I felt really lonely and lost. I loved being a mama, but I felt like I was losing a part of myself.

I stayed home with my babies for about eight years until I was ready to go back to teaching. Even then, I wasn't sure I was ready, but I knew I needed something for myself again.

I loved teaching at my new school. I learned a lot about myself over those years. My faith grew and so did my confidence. I felt like I was helping people. I learned I was good at teaching.

Teaching was a passion of mine, probably one I got from my mom who was also a teacher when I was growing up. Working at a faith-based school, I learned that your confidence can grow the more you help and serve others. I was surrounded by people who believed in me and lifted me up. Teaching was one of those experiences I needed to go through in order to see my gifts, which I would later use in other ways.

There is always a reason you go through a season or on a journey. You may not always understand it, but I promise you somewhere later down the road you will realize why your path was paved the way it was. Remember: life gives us blessings in disguise. Teaching taught me how to clearly communicate, how to speak in front of others and also to have empathy and compassion for them. I didn't realize it at the time, but this experience was preparing me for what was to come.

While I was teaching, I faced a number of challenging situations. Navigating interactions with private-school parents taught me the importance of speaking up for myself and setting clear boundaries to ensure I could thrive in a demanding environment.

It took me two years to start building my social media audience. I didn't know what I was doing, but since I loved makeup and teaching, I jumped right in recording my videos. The first mean comment I got devastated me. I laugh at it now, but at the time, I was in tears. The post was a family dance video where we would each dance to the camera as we listed our ages. When I danced to the front, the number 40 popped on the screen. Some guy, of course, who didn't follow me, commented I looked way older than 40. I felt completely defeated. I didn't have the skin of a twenty- year-old, but hey I was showing up!

As hard as those first comments were, I needed them. They kept me going even when sometimes I didn't want to post. The more I posted, the more mean comments I got, the more I learned to deal with them and realized that the person making those mean comments didn't have the confidence to show up like I was, so why did I care what they thought?

Confidence begins with your own opinion of yourself. Once you've decided that, no one else's opinion matters. Like we talked about in chapter six, being able to look in the mirror and accept what you see is more important than what anyone thinks of you. The more importance you place on what *you* think of you, the more your confidence grows and the less power others have to hurt your confidence.

As my social media grew, some amazing opportunities came my way. One of the coolest was making an appearance on Good Morning America. So many people in my corner were proud of me, cheering me on, and telling me I had made it. But I still didn't believe it. Even though I was building confidence in myself, I wasn't fully there yet. I wasn't celebrating my wins; I was focused on what was next. All I could see was what I hadn't accomplished yet — not where I was. Due to the lifelong drive to prove myself, I couldn't recognize my wins or believe that what I had done was "enough." But celebrating wins and accomplishments is part of building confidence. Think about how far you've come in life. Be proud of who you are now, so you can build the confidence to continue toward where you're going.

How Do I Build Confidence?

Here are some of the things I have learned along the ways that have helped me:

1. Stop comparing yourself to others. Someone is always going to do something different than you. Not better⊠ just different. We all have our own gifts; it is your job to find your gift and use it to help others. The more you compare or look at what others are doing, the more time you spend holding yourself back from shining. Stop trying to be like someone else and embrace who you are.

2. Celebrate and reflect on your wins. For some people this can be really hard. I never stopped long enough to see what I had accomplished. The small wins are as important as the large ones. Take time to be proud of yourself. You are evolving and changing and growing. Creating space to celebrate yourself and where you have come from will give you such a perspective switch,

and also make you be pretty damn proud of the new you!

3. Embrace your "failures" and view them as growth opportunities. There is no such thing as a failure in life. As I talked about in chapter three, "failures" are experiences you need to go through to get to where you are going. You are learning and growing and becoming a stronger version of you. Those little "blips" are experiences you must go through, so appreciate the journey.

4. Step out of your comfort zone. Just do it! Life is too short to sit back and be miserable. You can change your life at any time. It's a choice. You don't have to have the confidence or the experience. You just have to start. You just have to keep showing up until you realize you can do it. I believe in you, but you have to believe in yourself.

5. Have affirmation sessions. I am a big believer in affirmations and journaling. Affirmations teach you how to talk to yourself. Put your affirmations in places that you can see them every day. The bathroom mirror, your coffee pot, in your car, the regular places you look every day. This will reinforce your new thought process. Affirmations teach you to retrain your brain and how to see a new way, even when a positive outlook doesn't always seem possible. Some of my favorite affirmations are ones that are very simple: "I love who I am becoming," "I am brave," "Happiness is a choice," and "I am enough exactly as I am."

6. Pursue passions that make you happy! Listen, you are not stuck! You can pivot at any time and you can find your joy again. You just have to be brave enough to

try. What do you truly love to do? Do it! I love teaching and I loved teaching kids, but now I am just as equally passionate about helping women find their beauty and see their worth. I love teaching women that they are already enough. It is one of the most amazing feelings to see a woman feel beautiful in her skin again. When you follow your joy, you make an impact and change the world.

Confidence is a learned skill. The more you put yourself in uncomfortable positions, the more you will see growth and learn to trust yourself and your ability to do hard things. It's time to lean into the things that bring you joy. Lean into your gifts, because the world needs you to share them. The more you live out your passions, the more your confidence will grow and that confidence will impact everyone around you to find their confidence too.

Journal Questions

1. What are your strengths and how could you use them to build the life that you want?
2. What are your "wins?" When was the last time you celebrated something you have accomplished that you were proud of?
3. When was the last time you felt confident? What about that situation made you feel that way?

_____

_____

_____

_____

_____

_____

_____

_____

_____

_____

_____

_____

_____

_____

_____

_____

_____

_____

Makeup Mini-Tutorial: Applying Blush for Your Face Shape

As we age, gravity can take a toll in many ways on the face. Hollowing as well as loss of elasticity can cause the face to droop more than it used to. But did you know blush can change the look of your face? Check out this video and try some new techniques with your blush. You may find one you love!

https://www.instagram.com/p/C_b0VTav8P5/

Chapter Eight
Face It 'Til You Make It

Don't fake it till you make it. That's garbage advice. Face it till you make it. Get up. Work hard. Fail. Stand back up. Face it again. Do a little better. Fail again. Get back up. Repeat.

— Jordan Syatt

When I decided to start my social media accounts, I didn't know how to make an Instagram video. I didn't know what to say, let alone how to cut it or edit a video. I started off just talking about makeup issues I was personally struggling with and how I would fix them, but I honestly didn't know exactly what I was doing in the beginning. There were times I would use the wrong makeup on myself or color match a client with the wrong shade. But I had to start somewhere, so I continued to educate myself and learn the ins and outs of makeup and what would work on maturing skin.

I was scared. I was nervous and often embarrassed about what people would think of me. But I kept going. I showed up when

I didn't feel like it. I showed up when I didn't think anyone was watching. I showed up when it was hard. I just kept showing up—until one day, people started to notice.

I literally taught myself everything. I asked women my age what they struggled with when applying and wearing makeup and I wrote it all down. I made notes when women asked me questions about my makeup or voiced concerns on how their makeup was laying on their skin. I did research on what women over 40 were struggling with when wearing makeup, or why at 40 a lot of women stopped wearing makeup. I kept journals of the information I was learning and I started watching other videos and examining why they were getting a lot of likes and views. I made more notes.

Even before I started making an income, I invested in my business. I took classes on how to create content and how to apply makeup. I did makeup on women for free, so I could learn about how it applied on different skin types or how different face shapes required different methods. I hired business coaches. I took my new job seriously and I set goals for myself. I saw a future and even though I wasn't seeing success (yet), I put everything in place so that one day I would see all my hard work pay off.

After two years of making videos and doing lots of research I finally started to see growth. Could I have given up two years before and said that this wasn't for me. Could I have questioned if I was good enough? Could I have just quit? Of course! But I didn't. I buckled down and spent many late nights doing activities that would help me build the business I could see in my mind. I did all of this and also surrounded myself with people in my corner that wanted me to win.

I will never forget that after two years of really hard work and moving away from my teaching profession, one of my videos on makeup placement went viral. It was a simple video showing how I used to do my makeup when I was younger compared to how I do my makeup now in my forties. It outlined the placement of concealer, blush, and contour to show how makeup can age you or make you look younger. This video jump-started my account, and I quickly went from 20K followers to 170K followers in the matter of two weeks. It was crazy! I do free color matches for a makeup brand that I work for, and the number of matches coming in was insane. I was actually on a girls' weekend with a bunch of other women from the same makeup company the weekend that video went viral, and I will never forget them sitting down with me, laptops in hand, and helping me furiously color match. My eyes fill with tears thinking of that moment. I cannot believe how these women wanted me to win. I had finally found women who wanted to see me and my hard work succeed. After years of picking friends who didn't have my best interests at heart, witnessing a moment where I had finally found that was amazing. After struggling for years to show my authentic self and learning that it was okay to be me, I had found women who wanted to see me succeed.

That weekend was a blur, but I will never forget it because I was surrounded by women who saw my vision. If you can surround yourself with women who have the same goals and mindset as you, you can share ideas, collaborate and stay motivated toward achieving your goals. Having a community of people around you that lift you up on your hard days and cheers on your good ones reminds you that you're not alone and you can do hard things—it keeps you from giving up on your goals and dreams too early. And it gives you the chance to be the support for others as well.

When GMA contacted me to ask about appearing on a segment with them about how to help women over 40 age backward with makeup tips, I almost said no. Who was I to give advice? I literally asked myself that. I look back and laugh now! Thank goodness, despite my fear I said yes.

I had many calls with the producer before the show was set to be filmed at my house. My best friend agreed to be my model, which calmed so many of my fears. The woman I was when they filmed this segment was so naive. I had been filming on a tripod on my kitchen table in front of a window with no fancy equipment for the last two years. When *Good Morning America* showed up with their fancy lights and camera crew, my nervousness turned into fear. Everything became really real. This was out of my comfort zone!

The producer told me what to say and how to look at the camera correctly, making sure I had the right angles. Because of my nerves, I had to keep starting over and trying to remember my lines. Luckily they were so patient with me. My best friend, Chels, who was also my makeup model in the segment, kept trying to make me laugh and telling me to breathe. I truly believe without her there I wouldn't have enjoyed this moment.

I took a deep breath, and internally reminded myself I knew what I was talking about and finally leaned into myself. I knew how to teach and keep things easy, so I did it. It was like my body knew what to do and my words were flowing without me really knowing what I was exactly saying, but they were loving it.

Sometimes in these moments that take us so far out of our comfort zone we not only realize we can do hard things, but that we were meant to do them. This was one of these moments. I am forever grateful for it. I am grateful that I didn't follow my initial thought and say no when I was asked to do this segment because I didn't want to be uncomfortable. In hindsight, I laugh at how silly I was of being scared that I almost said no because I didn't think I could do it. It's funny how fear can make us think we can't do something. I am so grateful I didn't let fear hold me back from doing something that forever changed my trajectory in the social media world.

The segment aired about a week later and the amount of people happy for me was unreal. Sometimes when you are doing a job like mine, you feel pretty lonely. You are talking to a camera like it's your best friend and you often aren't even sure if someone is listening. The journey of going after something you want might be lonely. You might not always feel supported and you may question why you want something so bad, but when things start coming together you'll be surprised by who has always been in the background cheering you on even when you didn't expect it.

After my video went viral and *Good Morning America* featured me in a segment on their show, my account continued to gain more traction. I thought I had officially made it, but questioned myself for the next year. I didn't believe I was good enough to be this person on social media, so I sabotaged myself with self-doubt. No matter what you are doing, the doubt will come. No matter how much success you may see, until you decide you are good enough, that doubt can creep in.

Going after new goals or changing your life is going to come with ups and downs. There will be good, but there will also be some hard. Pushing yourself out of your comfort zone, puts us on a journey of self-growth. The good as much as the hard puts you on a journey of self-discovery. It teaches you to grow in ways you maybe never thought you could and the journey humbles you.

Keep Going Despite the Struggle

You are going to encounter struggles on your way to where you want to be. The problem isn't the hard parts— it's that most give up too early. They don't immediately succeed, so they give up. They walk away and they quit believing that winning is right around the corner.

It doesn't take a special person to hit goals. It takes someone who is downright determined. They know it won't be easy. They know they will make sacrifices and they know how much courage it takes to try something they aren't already good at. If you want to change your life, if you want to do something new, be ready for the struggle. Be ready to dig deep and be ready to work hard. Nothing comes easy, but the more you keep putting yourself out there, the more you will keep facing the hard and realizing that you are capable of more than you realized.

I know you may be in the thick of chasing your dreams right now, or maybe you want to start something but you're really scared. I want you to know, I've been there. I am still there! There are times I still question what I'm doing. Can we normalize that? We don't always know the struggles or pain someone went through in the beginning. That person you look up to...trust me they have struggles; you are just seeing their "end" story, but not where they truly began. No one starts anything knowing everything and everyone's journey and path is different.

Lean into not knowing. Follow your joy and let it take you for a ride. I promise you; you will learn a lot about yourself in the process. You will find your joy and live a fuller life than the person sitting in the background scared to start. Just by starting, you are facing the possibility of new life...of a new you.

Trust me, that old quote faking it till you make it...it doesn't work, because if you are faking it, you aren't being yourself. You aren't finding your joy. You are doing something to make someone else happy and you aren't leaning into your authentic self, which the world needs. Instead, face your fears until you do make it. The more you put yourself in uncomfortable situations the more you will learn that trying something new isn't really that scary. I believe in you, now it's time to start believing in yourself.

How to Change Your Path

Here are some things I did to change my career at 39 and pivot before I actually knew what I was doing:

1. I asked questions. Look at people who are doing what you want to do well. What are they doing? How can you make it your own (no copying, put your spin on it). Ask people in the industry you want to go into, how they got

started and their best advice. You are going to learn some valuable information when you start picking people's brains in your industry that are doing things well.

2. I leaned into my awkwardness. No one needs another copy of someone else. What are you good at? What makes you different from someone else? As I talked about in chapter six, lean into your authentic self, that is your superpower. No one is exactly you.

3. I did my research. How are others who are successful in your field doing it? YouTube, Google and watching what others are doing that is working for them can be really powerful.

4. I took baby steps and gave myself grace. You won't be perfect and no one knows what they are doing in the beginning. Like I stated in chapter three, you just have to start. You won't be good right away, you may be uncomfortable, but the hardest part is taking that first step and seeing that it isn't as scary as you thought.

5. I wrote myself affirmations. Put post-it notes around your house to remind you of who you are. Remind yourself of your why. Remind yourself that you are good enough and constantly keep these reminders where you can see them. There will be lots of times that you will need these reminders to keep going.

6. I educated myself. Take classes, practice and more practice. I used to ask friends to come over so I could practice my makeup skills on different face shapes and ages. It helped me see what worked and what didn't. I wasn't good at first, but the more I practiced, the better I got. Even when I was a teacher, college only prepared me a little bit. Once I got into an actual classroom was when I learned how to teach.

Journal Questions:

1. What is a new situation you are feeling unsure about starting?
2. What are your fears with this situation?
3. What is the worst thing that can happen by just starting? Best thing?

_____

_____

_____

_____

_____

_____

_____

_____

_____

_____

_____

_____

_____

_____

_____

_____

_____

_____

Makeup Mini-Tutorial: Lift Your Face

Makeup is like an art class. Shadows and applying darker colors in the wrong areas of the face can cause your face to look dark and droopy. Alternatively, using a light color can plump and give light to the face. This video will show you how using a lighter concealer color can lift and plump your face to make it appear more youthful. If you can make lines, you can start incorporating this trick into your makeup routine today!

https://www.instagram.com/p/DAzbEpkyrih/

Chapter Nine

Belief

Believe in yourself and all that you are. Know that there is something inside you that is greater than any obstacle.

— Christian D Larson

For many of us, the biggest dilemma we face is our own worst enemy: belief. We grow up loving who we are and believing we can do anything. But as we age, we start listening to others who tell us we can't do it, or that we aren't good enough. Pretty soon, those voices become louder than our own.

When I began working solely online, I couldn't have done it without others believing in me. My family, especially my husband, were my biggest cheerleaders. I got a lot of "no's" when I first started showing up. Brands didn't know me and people didn't trust me or want to buy any products. Contrary to what many people believe, you do not get paid for your follower account. So here I was, with very little income and I had just quit my stable teaching job.

I knew I needed a plan. I asked women to let me do their makeup for free if I could post a before and after photo. This gave me social proof. I asked women who tried the makeup brands I worked for to write testimonials about the product and how the makeup made them feel. I posted these online daily and this built credibility. The more I saw that others were believing in me, the more I believed in myself.

The women that I was helping sent me referrals. As my business grew, I focused solely on breaking down makeup in an easy educational way that women could understand and start having fun with makeup again. The more I saw women's faces light up and the more women started rediscovering their beauty, I realized I had found my gift. Sometimes it takes others to see your gift before you do. One of my best friends, who had been on social media longer than I had, saw my potential from the beginning. She helped mentor and guide me and was always cheering me on behind the scenes. Sometimes it takes lots of practice and doing the uncomfortable before you start believing in your gifts.

I was not the normal beauty content creator you see online. I was older and my skin was far from perfect, but women saw themselves in me. I was an average everyday mom of three teaching simple makeup tips to help makeup be fun again, and women started to support me because I was showing up as my true authentic self.

I also didn't know how to build a business. I remember spending Thanksgiving one year making my own website by following a YouTube tutorial, because I didn't have the money to pay someone to create it for me. I spent hours learning this new skill, late nights and early mornings, but I put the effort into bettering my business because I knew I could help others. I hired coaches, I watched my videos over and over again and critiqued them to make them better and easier to understand. I knew in order to believe in myself fully, I had to put the work in. I was able to put in the work, because I believed in myself. The work I did reinforced my belief.

I also gave myself lots of grace. I built belief in myself by being consistent. Consistency for me looked like doing things that kept me on track toward my goals. When you first begin working out, you have to start slow, but you have to continue to show up and do your exercises. If you skip the gym, or skip your walk even just for one day it can throw you off and even make you less likely to continue exercising. You have to make something a habit for it to stick. Likewise, I kept showing up on social media, even when no one else was cheering me on. Even when I got ten likes on a post, and when no one but my close family and friends were watching and supporting me, I kept going. It's really easy for your brain to tell you no one is supporting you or you aren't "good enough." Our brain wants to cling onto all the things we can't do and focus on that. It is our job to rewire our brain.

Violin Learnings

When I was in seventh grade, I decided to take up the violin. We didn't have a lot of money and I remember even the rent for the violin was more than my parents wanted to budget for.

My mom told me I could do it if I took it seriously, so the next thing I knew I was coming home with a shiny new violin in a big black case. I was really proud of that violin. I would carry it into school and home every day. I didn't ride the bus, so walking home from school wasn't always the easiest because that violin was heavy and I was tiny. After months of practicing, I felt like I was pretty good...however I would bet my family members would disagree. I think there was probably a lot of screeching and wrong notes being played, but hey, I was trying. That's how we all start out right? Trying! Showing up, putting the work in and building confidence in ourselves.

Every week, my violin teacher would have "play tests" during our orchestra test. We would have to stand up all by ourselves in front of everyone and play our part of the music we were learning. I hated them. Not only was I a very shy kid, I mean I would talk and my face would turn beat red, but standing up in front of a packed room of 50 kids and playing my violin was the absolute last thing I wanted to be doing. Based on how we played, we would then get placed in a "seat." This seat was basically a way to put the best players in the front and the worst players in the back. I dreaded every Friday, because I would get up and play my violin in a silent room and get so nervous that I would blank out and forget how to read the music on the page. Everything looked jumbled up and the room felt like it was spinning.

I usually ended up as the last seat in the violin section and that made me feel absolutely horrible. I felt like I sucked. I felt like giving up and I felt so defeated. Have you ever had times in life when you feel that way? The easy thing is to give up, right?

Well, that's what I wanted to do but my parents would not let me. They even got me violin lessons, which helped a little but I honestly don't think I was cut out to be a musician. I eventually quit playing the violin. I actually gave up the violin for a tennis racquet. I did give the violin a good go, but I never felt joy when I was playing. I often felt anxiety when I would have to practice or perform. This is a good lesson to remember too: You may not love everything you try, but trying new things helps you find your passions.

In hindsight, 30-something years later, I think my music teacher could have made a huge difference in my mindset and confidence by pulling me aside and offering some encouraging words and telling me what I was doing well instead of what I was always doing wrong. Maybe you haven't experienced a negative person in your life who doesn't see your worth, but it can be your own brain that is the one who is sending you constant messages that mess with your belief in yourselves. We are hardwired to see the negatives over the positives and if we cling to the negatives we will never build that belief in ourselves.

Belief and Failure

We lack belief because we are scared of failing. We are scared of not being good enough. We are scared of what others will think. When I say that out loud though, doesn't it sound silly? We limit ourselves from trying new things because we are worried about the future—when the future hasn't even happened yet!

Think of all the things you don't do in life because you are scared. I can name a few things I am deathly scared of—rollercoasters, heights, spiders, skiing. The list can get long. About two years ago, I decided to slowly start living more. I was going to push myself to do things I found that were hard for me or out of my comfort zone. One year I took a work trip with my girlfriends to Mexico. We visited a park that had a zipline that went through a tropical rainforest. It was incredibly beautiful, but I was set that I was not going to be able to do it. I was deathly scared of heights and this was high up in the treetops.

If it wasn't for my friends, I don't know if I would have made it through that day. They hyped me up, walked me through how it was going to feel and what to expect and told me to take it in baby steps. I went through the entire jungle and finished that zipline. I flew high up in the air through the trees screaming my heart out with joy. It was exhilarating, it felt freeing and to think I almost didn't get to experience it because I was almost too scared to try. Sometimes we let fear hold us back from trying new experiences because we tell ourselves it's something we can't do.

If you are struggling with belief, put people in your corner who want to see you succeed. The girls that walked me through the zipline experience that day will probably never know what an impact they had on me. They believed in me more than I believed in myself and sometimes we need that. The biggest lesson I learned is we don't have to conquer everything at once—it's the baby steps that get us where we want to be. They build our beliefs. With each step, we begin to believe in ourselves and are willing to take one step more—pretty soon we have climbed our huge mountain of disbelief and end up believing that we can do the things we didn't believe we could.

The Power of Affirmations

Another way to "remind" yourself who you are and what you want is to see what you want. Have a vision and write it down. A couple of years ago, when I was seriously doubting what I was doing, I was depressed and showing up on social media was the last thing I wanted to do.

I felt like no one wanted to support me or even watch the content I was creating, which, for me, meant my income wasn't growing. My husband took it upon himself to remind me of my worth. During this time, we started watching *Ted Lasso*, a show all about belief. One night, I went to bed early, and when I woke up the next morning, there were yellow post-it notes all over the house. He had placed a yellow post-it with the word BELIEVE in every corner I might go to: the bathroom mirror, inside the fridge, the doors of the house, my nightstand... everywhere. He also wrote affirmations like "You are brave," "You are allowed to be powerful," "I value my opinions over anyone else's," and, my personal favorite, "I don't need to impress others; I only seek validation from myself" on my mirrors in dry erase markers. He told me to read them every day, and even though I didn't believe in myself yet, the more I read the notes, the more I began to believe I could do the hard things. He also often reminded me to 'be a goldfish.' Why a goldfish? Because goldfish don't get offended; they move on fast and forget quickly.

He was right. It wasn't an instant fix, but it kept me going and things started to change. My body language became more confident. Instead of moping around the house focusing on things I couldn't control, I focused on the things I could control, like how I treated others, how I started my day with a good routine and talking to myself in an intentional and positive way. I began believing the affirmations I was reading and changing my thought patterns.

Rewiring my brain to think differently and to believe in what I was doing changed how I showed up online. Instead of thinking about the things I wasn't good at, or focusing on what wasn't happening for me, I would say things like, "I choose to believe in myself no matter what is happening around me." "The universe is for me." "I have a lot to bring to the table." These affirmations taught me that belief does not happen overnight, but focusing on the small steps brings you to where you want to be. It also taught me to trust that anything is possible. Trust and see it, even when it isn't happening. The vision is what spurs your belief.

How to Believe in Yourself

So how do you believe in yourself, even when you aren't getting results? Here is what I did:

I kept showing up online even when I didn't know what I was doing and I got a lot of "no's". I had people ghost me or not answer me. When my following was still small, brands didn't want to work with me, so I started showing and talking about products I loved because I knew being genuine was better than talking about products I didn't really love just for clout or payment. I remained true to myself and stayed authentic.

Building my makeup business and earning an income from selling makeup was challenging and really difficult. It was tough in the beginning when people were just watching me but not trying the makeup. I knew I had to gain trust. Think of the things you buy online, right? You don't always buy the product, you are buying it because you respect and trust the person or even friend who is telling you about it. So, I asked women to post before and after photos of their makeup after they tried it. I asked them to write up what the makeup was doing for them, how I had helped them. They sent me referrals. I posted testimonials and started breaking down educational content that helped women start to actually understand makeup.

Starting and growing my business was hard and money was tight. I couldn't afford to hire assistants to help me with the workload, so I watched hours of YouTube videos trying to figure out how to make my own website. I asked lots of questions from people in my industry that were more experienced than me. I asked questions about how they got started, what they were doing that was working for them, how they were using automations in their business, or how they learned how to use different websites to list products they were talking about. I watched how other successful content creators showed up on stories and what they were doing in their videos. I watched body language, hooks they were using and even researched hashtags. I watched my own videos and critiqued them over and over to make them better and easier to understand. As I got farther along in my business, I used systems to help run my business more efficiently. My belief in myself that I could do hard things grew every time I figured something else on my own.

All the hard work and all the struggling to figure things out on my own built my belief in myself. Every time I accomplished something I didn't think I could do, but did it, my belief would grow. I leaned on this belief I was building often throughout my first couple years, because I started to doubt myself the bigger my account grew and the more success I found. As my business grew, I was able to hire coaches to teach me how to position myself in front of a camera and how to film catchy videos, which in turn helped me create better content, reach more people, and grow the business even more. Learning from others and having them critique what I was doing helped me be more intentional when making content. I started creating content in a different way and my following count grew, which grew my belief in myself. I was attracting like-minded women to my account who were loving the things I was teaching and sharing!

I think it is important to add that no matter how strong your belief is in yourself, there will be times that belief will waver. Imposter syndrome may creep in. You may ask yourself, "Who am I to be doing this?" This is normal! The key is to build a strong foundation and having anchors to remind yourself of your belief when you begin to doubt. Whenever I felt my belief waver, I would read my affirmations and lean on the people who were cheering me on. I also kept encouraging messages from women that followed me and had reached out to tell me why they loved following me. It sounds silly, but those messages got me through so many times that I wanted to quit. Putting people in your corner that want you to win and can remind you of why you are making a difference is so important when you waiver in your belief in yourself.

The more inner work you do to build yourself up, the easier it will be to bounce back when life gets hard, because it will. Especially as a business owner. You will have ups and downs. As an influencer on social media, I often feel like I am on a rollercoaster. People will love me one week and hate me the next. And when the haters are out, they make sure to tell me how wrong I am. Even now, it can be downright hurtful.

Learning that people usually attack you because of their own traumas and standing true in your belief in yourself is what gets you through when others try to put you down. Your opinion is the only one that matters.

This is true in life too. Even the other day, my daughter and I were having our picture taken at a gathering at a friend's house. I looked over and one of the moms and her daughter were whispering and laughing while looking at us. This would have bothered me years ago and I would have been so hurt, wondering what I was doing to make them talk about us. Instead, because I know who I am and what I stand for, I didn't think twice. Nothing others do is because of you. It took me a long time to build that belief in myself. It took years of being treated wrongly by women, to understand how I wanted and deserved to be treated. Be strong in who you are, what others do has nothing to do with you. Stand in your truth and others will see your light and want more of it.

Building a belief in yourself takes time. It won't happen overnight. Give yourself lots of grace as you navigate and the journey of building that belief. You can learn to change your belief system. Taking time to examine your current beliefs and deciding if you want to believe those things is how you start to change them. You can change it at any time. It is a mindset shift. Once you start to see your gifts and what you have to offer, you will realize that no one but you has the ability to be you. Knowing who you are and what you have to offer can only be done when you know who you are and what you believe. That is your superpower.

Journal Questions

1. When you have doubted yourself, how did you handle those moments?
2. How do you react to criticism or feedback, and what does that tell you about how you believe in yourself?
3. How do you think you can give yourself grace and find compassion as you build self-belief?

Makeup Mini-Tutorial: Lip Liner Tips

If you notice your lips have lost the volume, they once had, you are not alone! Unless you're using filler, there are not many ways to plump and create fuller lips. This trick will give the illusion of a fuller lip with just a lip liner and a lipstick or gloss.

https://www.instagram.com/p/C8mbYKHJ7w8/

Chapter Ten

You Haven't Lost Yourself

Aging is out of your control, how you handle it though, is in your hands.

— Diane Von Furstenberg

A lot changed for me in the summer of 2023. My body didn't feel like my own. I was feeling really anxious, alone and depressed. My body was changing. Despite working out and healthy eating habits, I was gaining weight around the midsection. My brain felt like it didn't work. I had always been someone who could make an imaginary list in my head and remember everything, and now I couldn't even remember my neighbor's name. It felt like early onset dementia, but I was only 42.

I didn't want to be around anyone. My moods were out of control. I found myself yelling and screaming at my husband or kids for the silliest things. Road rage became a real thing and my moods were like a rollercoaster. Happy, to sad, to angry in less than a couple of minutes.

My joints hurt and I can't even tell you how many doctors' appointments and physical therapy appointments I went to for my shoulder pain. I lost range of motion and could hardly move it about my head. It hurt to sleep at night as every time I rolled over I winced in pain.

Talk about sleepless nights...I would dread going to bed. The clock next to my bed would hit 3:00 a.m., my internal alarm clock would go off, and I would be awake for the rest of the night. My nights would consist of endless worry and night anxiety about things I couldn't control. I would worry if I was being a good enough parent. I worried about my job and if I would be able to make a good enough income that month. I worried that the doors were all locked in the house and the list of endless worries grew the more days I didn't sleep.

One night, I had a panic attack so bad I sat up in bed crying endlessly while my husband tried to console me. I was screaming and crying and felt so out of control. I knew something was wrong, but I didn't know what.

Not long after, I was talking to my mom on the phone and she straight up told me to go to a doctor. She told me she thought my hormones were off and I needed help. I'm not honestly sure why I listened to her. I am stubborn when it comes to going to a doctor. Up until that point, even though my husband is a physician assistant, I had steered clear from doctors. I didn't like going because I didn't like finding out something could be wrong with me. I know I went this time, because I was fed up with being an emotional rollercoaster, but I went.

Before I keep going with this story, I want you to know that if you can relate to any of this you are not alone. This was one of the loneliest and low points of my life and to be honest I have never felt more alone.

My husband's attending physician is a functional medical doctor who worked at the Mayo Clinic and specializes in women's hormones. I didn't know this was a big deal at the time, but it was. What I learned when I went to see Dr. Willey was that I was going through something called perimenopause.

Perimenopause wasn't a very talked about subject, even a year ago. It wasn't something that I had heard any of my friends talking about and I had no clue what it even was when I was diagnosed. Even a year later, I feel like more women are starting to speak up now, but at the time not many were. Women like Dr. Mary Claire Haver have paved the way for more education and research on this topic and so many more women are becoming aware of what it is. Perimenopause is a stage of life when estrogen and progesterone levels begin to fluctuate. It typically starts in your 40s, but some women enter it as early as 35. Perimenopause can last seven to ten years and is the stage before menopause. Many women have symptoms like night sweats, hot flashes, anxiety, hair loss, mood changes, brain fog, weight gain and more. There are over 40 symptoms of perimenopause and I was experiencing quite a few of them.

Most women report the worst symptoms around the age of 42. I am sure a lot of us are experiencing them earlier, but for some reason they become unbearable in our early 40s for many of us. Many women report that it just feels like their spark is gone. I could truly relate.

When I sat down with Dr. Willey, I felt crazy. I felt like he was going to think I was making all of this up, but he didn't. He actually listened. I unleashed all of my issues, all of my frustrations on him while he just listened. It made me feel less crazy. When I was all done he told me I was normal. My hormones were out of balance and he had a plan.

I was blessed that I had found a functional medicine doctor. When most women see their family practice doctor or OBGYN, they're sent away saying their bloodwork is normal and it's all in their head. The interesting thing about perimenopause and women's hormones are very individualized. When functional medical physicians are looking at hormone levels, they should be driven by symptoms. An estradiol level can be within range but not at an optimal level for someone. Checking FSH levels versus blood tests are often much more reliable when determining if someone is in perimenopause.

I didn't know that the day I saw Dr. Willey would change my life and the trajectory of my 40s. I knew other women were feeling that same isolation I was going through. So many women are struggling in silence. For many of us, our bodies are changing. There aren't many answers on the internet and finding a doctor who understands women's hormones is often hard.

Because this was something nobody talks about and finding answers is so hard, I felt called to share my journey with other women, so one day I shared a video. In that video, I showed all the frustrations I had been experiencing with perimenopause. Weight gain, changes in my face and body, endless supplements, brain fog and loneliness. The video went viral and so many women were telling me they felt seen. I knew my story needed to be told.

Why am I so passionate about talking about perimenopause and my journey with it? I think mostly because my mother's generation was taught to be silent. I also am not sure that many women of my mother's generation even knew what perimenopause was or what was happening with their bodies—just that they were getting older. Menopause has been something that has gotten more attention since it is easier to mark with period loss. I am so thankful for my mom realizing I needed to be seen by a doctor. Many women don't know what to do and depression sinks in. I also look at my fifteen-year-old daughter and never want her to be silent about her body. I never want her to not understand her body, so I share because of her too.

I love this quote by Cherie Fournier, a perimenopause blogger: "Perimenopause is a fact of life. There's no need to cover up what's happening with our minds and bodies to minimize it or to be ashamed of it." So many of us were taught growing up to be quiet; to not talk about our bodies and I honestly think that is why so many of us are accepting that this is the way our new life will be. Perimenopause is not a disease. Our hormones are changing. Perimenopause affects every woman in one way or another, even if their symptoms look different.

The day I went to see Dr. Willey, he listened. He gave me solutions and we are working together to educate other women on perimenopause. So many women every year are sent away by doctors telling them this is normal and you just have to get through it. Women walk away feeling lost. The truth is there is so much that women can do during this time and feel supported.

Because I was encouraged to get help, I encourage women every day to keep searching for answers, and find someone who will listen to them. Fighting for better treatment and care is so important, as is telling your own story. Start talking about it. Talk to your girlfriends and your daughters and share your experiences. This is what will help us all through this time. We women are going through so many changes, and going through it alone and suffering in silence is unnecessary.

How to Manage Perimenopause Symptoms

There are so many things you can do if you feel this way too.

If you are experiencing weight gain, moving your body in small ways can make a big difference. My functional medical doctor suggested taking a walk after my last meal of the day without my phone and enjoying the world around me. Not only is this good for weight loss, but it is also great for your mood. Even if you have never been to the gym before, find a yoga class or go for walks around the block; start slow by making new habits. Lifting weights is also important for bone density. We lose muscle as we age and this will help build and keep you strong. It will also boost your metabolism.

Eat a diet rich with protein. Look into anti-inflammatory foods like fish, leafy greens, avocados and walnuts. I included many of these into my diet and also did a lot of research on Keto and Mediterranean diets. I tried many of them and they didn't always work for me. For example, the Keto diet actually had me starving and I gained weight not having carbs. For some people it will work though, so there is definitely not a one size fits all when it comes to finding a meal plan that works for you. One way of eating doesn't work for everyone.

You may need to experiment with different foods and eating plans to find the one that resonates with your body. After meeting with my functional medicine physician, we discussed various supplements that could help alleviate my perimenopause symptoms. During this time, I was feeling extremely anxious, and he prescribed ashwagandha and boswellia. He also discussed peptides with me. Peptides are supplements that contain peptides that naturally occur in the body. I have a long list of the supplements I have taken and am taking on my website at laurenhalebeauty.com. Always consult with your physician before taking any supplements, as I am obviously not a trained medical professional, just someone trying to navigate perimenopause.

Next, make sure to find a doctor who will listen. I personally suggest a functional medical physician who specializes in women's hormones. Many doctors do not get the training for women's hormones in residency and a blood test is not all that is needed to diagnose you with perimenopause. A functional medical doctor will listen to your symptoms first, look at your medical history, and your age. They will also ask about your menstrual cycle, and yes you can still have a period and be in perimenopause. They will also usually do a blood test as well, but it is not the only factor. There are no normal results. Everyone is different and the right physician will take into account all of the factors I stated above before making a diagnosis. Think back to when we all hit puberty or started our periods, it wasn't at the same time right? We don't experience our period in the same way or start at the exact same time as someone else so it is important to remember that our bodies are different, our history is different and we don't all go into perimenopause at the same time or experience it in the exact same way either.

Find support. Lean on your girlfriends, husbands or anyone who is willing to listen. I have built a large community of women encouraging and supporting each other on social media on Instagram so come find me over there if you need some extra encouragement too! Give yourself grace as you navigate the changing symptoms and know not every day will be easy. Take it day by day and be proud of yourself and your body—it can do hard things.

Explore your options. There are so many choices out there for women now. Hormone replacement and supplements have changed my life. They may not be options for you, but ask your doctor questions. Be your biggest advocate and get a second opinion if you need one. The research and options have changed and developed in huge ways since our parents' generation.

Lastly, remember you are not lost, there are ways to find your joy again. What used to bring you joy? Try and remember back to those things and do more of it. For me, it was taking time for myself again. For years, I was wrapped up in the identity of being only a mom. I would plan play dates, be the school mom, or be unavailable at night because it was bath time. Now that my kids are older and don't need me like they once did, I am trying to find time for myself again and remember what I used to love to do. Going to the gym, taking a bubble bath every night, and traveling with my husband, those things remind me that I still matter. Finding the things that bring you joy will help you find yourself again. It will help you remember that you have purpose. It will teach you to age gratefully rather than focus on what you feel your body can't do right now. Sometimes being in perimenopause can feel like our bodies aren't ours anymore, so focusing on the things we can control during this time is so important so that we don't hyperfocus on all the changes we are experiencing.

You aren't the same as you once were when you were younger. You have changed and you are in the process of finding out who you are again. Give yourself grace. Give your body grace—it has been through a lot. Know that you may not know who you are right now, but you will find that person again. Keep fighting to get your sparkle back. Keep fighting to find *you* again.

Journal Questions

1. What brings you joy or what used to bring you joy? How can you do more of that?
2. What are some healthy habits you can start implementing today?
3. What are you most proud of yourself for?

_____

_____

_____

_____

_____

_____

_____

_____

_____

_____

_____

_____

_____

_____

_____

_____

_____

_____

_____

_____

Makeup Mini-Tutorial: You Are Going Through Perimenopause

This video was a real and raw post for me. One of my kids is a senior in high school, and all of my kids were in or entering into their teenage years, and I felt a little lost as a mom. Add perimenopause into the mix and it was a perfect storm. Whether you have children or not, or whether your kids are young or old, I think most can relate to this post. Every stage and every chapter of life is a new one that we have navigated before and the changes that come may not always be ones we are ready to embrace. I hope this video, wherever you are in your life, helps you feel less alone.

https://www.instagram.com/p/C2qjW2EPwp4/

Chapter 11

You are Enough

Perhaps when you thought you weren't good enough, the truth was you were overqualified.

— Unknown

I've been a go-getter my whole life. When I took up tennis at thirteen, I even pictured myself playing on the courts at Wimbledon one day. I would sit and watch my tennis idols for hours. I analyzed what they were doing, watched interviews, read their biographies and dreamed about my turn. Now my journey didn't quite end up at that level, but I did secure myself a D I tennis scholarship when no one thought that was possible. We didn't have a lot of money, so I spent hours working at the local country club in order to pay for court time. I also had a lot of coaches notice my hard work and offer me free coaching sessions. I never once questioned that I couldn't do something I put my mind to.

Once I got to college, I think my eyes were opened when I saw these amazing girls who had been playing since they were three years old hitting the ball harder than I had ever even seen. It was intimidating. This was the first time I started really doubting myself and what I was doing.

This doubt would start plaguing me throughout my adult life. It's crazy how our minds are so powerful. I was around other women and the stories they told themselves started affecting me.

Most of us were raised hearing a particular story about ourselves. The people around you had a major impact on how your brain processed your surroundings. You may not remember doubting yourself until you got older, or maybe you remember from a young age comparing your body and abilities to someone else's.

Growing up in the 80s and 90s we were inundated with TV shows and magazines showing us women what a perfect body should be or what "sexy" looked like. Even if you weren't allowed to have those magazines in your house, you saw them in the grocery store or at a friend's house. I know I did! I remember women on a man-driven talk show being weighed on a scale or being told they were too big, when they were a size that was so small. We watched this. We grew up being told we were less-than.

In college, I was in a relationship with a guy I really liked. He was also a tennis player and for the first time in my life, I changed everything about who I was to be liked by him. It was never enough and eventually he cheated on me with another girl. After we broke up, I was devastated. I thought I would be more attractive if I was thinner, so I stopped eating. My love for tennis went away and I had no desire to do anything. Looking back,

I lost a lot in that relationship. I lost who I was. I was willing to be something I wasn't for someone else just to be liked. I ended up in the hospital needing IVs because I was so dehydrated from surviving on saltine crackers. I thought if I could just change myself, that guys would like me more. The stress of that relationship was one that I would deal with for years to come. This was another reason I walked away from my tennis career a year later, because I was so depressed and lost.

Hiding Behind Success

When I walked away from my identity as a tennis player, it was the first time I didn't know what I wanted to do in life. I was stuck on the identity I had created for myself and was embarrassed and ashamed that I had walked away from everything I had known, but my love for the game was gone.

The more I played up my successes, the more they became my identity and the more they became my identity, the more I focused on not failing. This message played over and over in my head, until all I heard was, *I am not good enough.* I learned to be tough on the inside and hide how I was feeling. I was good at not letting people get too close to me and hid my feelings, so it looked like nothing was ever bothering me. This helped me in sports, but lost me a lot of friendships and relationships because I was good at hiding behind my feelings and had a hard time letting anyone in.

This led to many years of having a tough exterior and hiding my emotions. I became really good at hiding behind the mask of happiness even though I didn't always feel this way. That tough exterior was a hard one for many to chip and I struggled with my friendships a lot during this time.

At just twenty-one years old, I started the long journey of finding myself again, even though at that young age I had no clue that's what I was doing. It took until my late 30s to finally start loving myself for the first time in my life. Navigating motherhood as a young mom with three kids and learning how to be a good communicator and wife to my husband were just two of the struggles I went through. I was so full of doubt for so long, even though on the outside my life looked perfect.

As I got older, I realized I never stopped to celebrate my accomplishments. I was too worried about making everyone happy around me. Too busy hitting my goals, that I never stopped to celebrate what I had done. I was too busy climbing the mountain to my next goal that I never appreciated the mountain I had just climbed. If you can relate, you know that this can become an endless and tireless journey of never thinking you have done anything.

In a world full of people and messages telling you aren't beautiful enough, you aren't smart enough, you can't do something good enough...the reality is you start believing it. As an overachiever, I strived for recognition. I loved telling everyone my accomplishments, but deep down (and years later) I realized I was hiding my insecurities behind these stories. I wanted people to like me, to fit in, to be noticed.... don't we all.

Fast forward to my 40s and starting this new life on social media. My daughter had just entered her teens and at the time I was on a healing journey to figure out what was important for me to feel accomplished. I realized that the only way I would stop and even be a little excited about my accomplishments was if someone recognized me. I was relying on others to see my worth, instead of me recognizing that these accomplishments had nothing to do with my worth. Those accomplishments had become my identity.

It wasn't until I decided I was tired of hiding behind all of this that I started to work on healing myself. I had to learn to be vulnerable. I had to learn to stop people pleasing. I actually had to have real conversations = not just with myself, but others. I had to learn to allow myself to feel my emotions, something I was never quite able to do growing up.

In a way, my newly teenage daughter was my inspiration. She was so innocent and her zeal for life was something I never wanted her to lose. Because of her, I made a choice to stop letting others live my life for me and instead live for myself. I was exhausted from living for others and their opinions. I spent my days journaling, repeating affirmations and digging into my past to figure out why my thought patterns were the way they were.

I stopped trying to be perfect. I was imperfectly perfect, we all are! I realized that you can't ever accept that you are enough if you don't love yourself. There is no need to put effort into yourself, because you already are enough. Instead of striving for more, I started realizing I already was everything I was supposed to be.

Being on social media hasn't been easy. The noise can be loud. I wasn't going to be for everyone and honestly that has been hard. The people pleaser in me wanted to be liked, but the fact is the more I worked on myself, the more I didn't care. I was tired of wanting to be everything for everyone and wanted to instead find the people that loved me for who I already was.

You Are Enough, Always

A couple years ago, I found a "You Are Enough" bracelet on Etsy and it became my life's motto. I actually never take this bracelet off because it is my constant reminder that no matter what I do, I will always be enough. No matter what someone says to me, I am already enough and so are you. It is a truth I want every woman to see in herself.

Success isn't an outside perspective. My husband's best piece of advice is something he always says to me: "Trust the process, not the outcome." When I'm doubting myself it really helps refocus on the moment. You don't have to put any effort into being good enough, because you already are. Your journey is going to have ups and downs, but your happiness is found within the journey. It's important to not be overly focused on your end goal. Stay focused on the present and all the little wins you have in the moments leading up to your ultimate goal, which is remembering who you are. You are a queen, so hold your head up high and start showing up as the person you are!

Learning to embrace who you are, including the parts you don't find perfect, is true acceptance. You already are enough; it just takes you believing that you have something to offer the world that no one else does. Once you remember that, sharing those parts of you will allow other women to truly shine too.

There will also always be days that you don't feel enough. Listen, this is normal. You have a bad day, your hormones are surging out of control, someone says something that triggers you....NORMAL! It's all about how fast you can get back in tune to you, that's what's important. Those triggering situations happen for your benefit. They test how far you've come and how you learn to let go. Here are some affirmations I love to use when I'm having a day where I don't feel good enough:

- You are all you need to be.
- You are sufficient.
- You are exactly where you should be.
- The things that are meant for you will find you.

By repeating these affirmations, you stop focusing on what you are lacking and instead find yourself in a grateful headspace. Being grateful helps you celebrate your successes and growth and still gives you the ability to always know there is more you can do tomorrow.

Journal Questions

1. What are 3 things you appreciate about yourself?
2. Write down some statements you say that are negative toward yourself. Now counter them with a positive statement that challenges those thoughts. For example, "I can't do makeup." Counter: "I am really coachable when learning new skills."
3. What are three accomplishments you want to celebrate in your life?

_____

_____

_____

_____

_____

_____

_____

_____

_____

_____

_____

_____

_____

_____

_____

_____

Makeup Mini-Tutorial: Steal My Genius Eyeshadow Tips

In this video, you'll see the easiest eyeshadow tips that anyone can use—no matter your eye shape or age. I hope you walk away from this video ready to conquer some new eye looks. This video gives my top tips for how to achieve the perfect (and simple) eye look.

https://www.instagram.com/p/C92uUGevOlx/

Conclusion

Unlocking Your Greatness

Wherever you are, at whatever age, you're only a thought away from changing your life.

— Wayne Dyer

I hope since reading this book, you've found joy again. Joy in embracing aging and all the changes that come with it. We are constantly learning more about ourselves and I hope by sharing my story about overcoming my lack of belief, it can spur you to remember that little girl inside of you that once believed in herself too.

My hope is that this book will help you rewrite the story of your past and give you the push you need to embrace your future and start living the life you want and going after the dreams you have had since you were little. Those dreams are possible. It's time to stop sitting back and letting life just pass by, and start living the life that you want.

I hope that by sharing my struggles, you can also see that anything is possible. We are constantly rewriting our stories.

It takes one simple yes to change your life. Letting go of all the things that have been holding you back, isn't just freeing—it is life changing. Life is too short to live your entire life not going after the things you want.

This book is a guide to coming back to yourself. To embrace who you have become, the mistakes, the highs and the lows have all brought you here. It's time to stop clinging to fear and old beliefs and time to try something new. It's time to live for yourself instead of others.

Growing older is a gift not many get to live. What are you doing to fully live it? Start sharing your stories, start being loud and start being okay with shining bright. You are uniquely you and the world needs you. Life is too short to sit back and hope things happen for you. Go after your dreams, tell people you love them, and share your gifts because no one else is you. It's time to start living now.

The key principles I have talked about in this book are all ones that have helped me grow stronger as a person. I truly believe that sharing our experiences teaches us that vulnerability is strength. None of us is perfect. We haven't lived a life without mistakes, but those "mistakes" have taught us more about life than anything else.

Embrace the messiness and start loving who you are. Confidence starts with how you feel about yourself and that is a choice. It's a mindset switch. You have the choice to start right now. Embracing this new chapter of your life and finding your joy again can happen.

I hope after reading this book, you realize that you are enough. You have ALWAYS been enough. Life is out there waiting for you; it's your job to go live it.

If you would like to connect with me, please follow me as I continue to navigate aging and share my story. I would love for you to watch my journey and message me about yours too. You can find me on Instagram, Facebook, YouTube and TikTok @ laurenlhale.

Here is the link to subscribe to my newsletter where I share all of my monthly favorite things, my family life and wisdom I am learning along the way too.

https://notable-mouse-168.myflodesk.com/fyx9y3oq2j

Here's What To Do Next

1. Connect with me on social media!
Follow me on all my social media platforms! You can find me on all social channels @laurenlhale.

2.Subscribe to my email list so you can find more inspiration and all the things I share
https://notable-mouse-168.myflodesk.com/fyx9y3oq2j.

3. Hire me to speak

If you are looking for a motivational speaker for your conference, event, or mastermind, I'd love to bring it!

Email <u>lauren.hale2@gmail.com</u> with "SPEAKING" in the subject line.

Acknowledgments

I want to thank my amazing husband, the love of my life, for always being my biggest cheerleader, best friend, support system and overall biggest fan. Without you, I wouldn't be where I am today. You are the one that tells me to chase my dreams and believe in myself, oftentimes more than I believe in myself.

To my children, thank you for teaching me more about who I am. Thank you for loving me even when I am imperfect. I wrote this book for you, so that one day when you doubt yourself you can remember your true potential comes from within.

To my mom and dad- thank you for teaching me that life is full of abundance. Thank you for teaching me to never give up and for allowing me to live my dreams. You always put me first and never questioned what I wanted to do. You just supported me. I hope that I can be that way always with my own kids.

Thank you to the staff at Grace Lutheran School for teaching me about faith. For instilling in me what family means, and for loving me unconditionally. The memories I had within those school walls are ones that truly molded me into who I have become.

Thank you to one of my best friends, Chelsea. You believed in me before I ever believed in myself. You saw potential in me before I knew it existed. Who knew a makeup palette could bring such a great friend into my life, when I really needed one. Thank you for always being that patient friend who never leaves my side.

To one of my biggest confidants, Taylor: Thank you for being that listening ear. The one who is always rational and who helped me through some tough years when I didn't know how I would get through. Thank you for questioning me and always making me question life. Your friendship is one I hold very close.

Lastly, to the coaches, teachers, friends who have come and gone, coworkers and mentors that I have had throughout my life: I would not be here without you. You all taught me lessons I needed to learn in order to become the best version of myself and for that I am grateful.

About the Author

Lauren Hale is a kindergarten teacher turned mature beauty influencer. Her goal is to teach women over 40 how to make their make-up work for their needs—instead of trying to make their skin work with the trends from 20-year-olds. She has over 800k followers on her social media platforms, and her work has been featured on *Good Morning America*, the *New York Post*, and the *Daily Sun*.

She lives in Idaho with her best friend and husband, Nic, and their three teenagers, who keep them busy traveling all over the northwest for a truly astounding number of sports tournaments. (And she wouldn't have it any other way.)

You can find her on Instagram, TikTok, or YouTube at @laurenlhale, or visit her website at laurenhalebeauty.com.

Made in the USA
Coppell, TX
08 July 2025

51601147R00094